Kripalu Yoga:
Meditation-in-Motion

Revised & Enlarged Edition

by

Yogi Amrit Desai

Second Edition
Second Printing, 1985
Third Printing, 1990
All Rights Reserved
Copyright 1981, 1984
by Kripalu Yoga Fellowship

Library of Congress Catalog Card Number: 85-80754
ISBN: 0-940258-11-0

Printed in the United States of America
by Kripalu Publications
P. O. Box 793
Lenox MA 01240

NOTE: This volume incorporates material from the 1981
booklet *Kripalu Yoga: Meditation-in-Motion*, published
by Kripalu Publications.

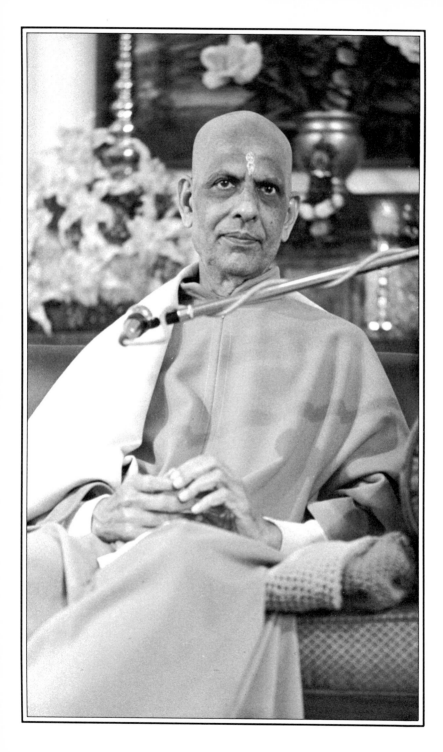

Dedicated in loving memory
of my Gurudev,

Swami Shri Kripalvanandji

whose love and grace
awakened within me
the living life force—prana—
that transformed my life,
and for whom I have named
this new dimension of yoga.

"Just as the purpose of Zen archery
is not merely to hit the target;
the purpose of the martial arts
not just to overcome the enemy;
and the purpose of koans
not merely to find
the answer to a question;
so also in Kripalu Yoga,
the purpose of the practice of asanas
is not merely to perfect the postures
or their physical benefits,
but rather to use them as a tool
to transcend the limitations
of the ego-mind,
and to awaken
to our highest potential."

—Yogi Amrit Desai

Table of Contents

Preface

This volume is the first to appear about Kripalu Yoga, a radically new approach to the traditional practice of classical yoga, developed by Yogi Amrit Desai.[1]

In it, Yogi Desai describes for the first time the extraordinary personal experience he had in 1970 that gave birth to Kripalu Yoga. He describes how one morning during his daily yoga practice he unexpectedly entered into an ecstatic state of expanded consciousness, during which his body began to perform yoga postures automatically and spontaneously.

At that point he had spent over twenty years mastering and teaching the art of traditional Ashtang yoga,[2] was founder and director of one of the largest yoga societies in America (which graduated over 2000 students every semester), and was widely regarded and honored as an authority on yoga both in India and

FOOTNOTES

[1]This technique is already being practiced and taught in many countries around the world and is widely recognized as an authentic new approach to classical yoga. Each year over the last ten years nearly 100 new Kripalu Yoga teachers have graduated from the Kripalu Center for Yoga and Health in Lenox, Massachusetts, founded by Yogi Desai and now one of the largest and most highly reputed centers of its kind in the country, with a resident staff of over 250.

[2]The classical eight-step system, comprising hatha and raja yogas. Hatha yoga consists of physical disciplines, such as postures and breathing exercises; raja yoga consists of mental disciplines, such as concentration and meditation.

in the United States. Yet his profound experience in 1970 totally revolutionized everything he thought he knew about yoga and brought a depth of insight and joy to his practice that he had not suspected possible.

He recognized that this experience, which he termed "Meditation-in-Motion," was the result of what yogis call "the awakening of *prana*, (the intelligent life force within us)."[3] The prana thus freed in his body, together with his deep understanding of and insight into its workings, radically transformed not only his whole perception and practice of yoga, but also every facet of his life.

In contrast to the unpredictability usually reported about such "peak experiences," he found he was able to enter into this meditative consciousness again and again at will during his daily yoga practice. By studying the causative principles behind these experiences, he was able to develop from them a whole new approach to the practice of yoga so that anyone can enter into similar experiences of Meditation-in-Motion and personal transformation.

Kripalu Yoga is a unique, five-stage system in which postures (hatha yoga) are used as a medium for inducing mental disciplines (raja yoga) by consciously using the intelligence of prana. Each stage is planned to progressively prepare both the body and mind to help awaken prana. Thus Kripalu Yoga is a new ap-

---

[3]The awakening of prana is an integral part of what is more commonly known as kundalini awakening.

proach where both the hatha and raja yoga phases of Ashtang yoga and the prana awakening principles of Kundalini yoga are incorporated simultaneously as one holistic practice.

Traditionally, Ashtang yoga is practiced as the path of will, in which movements of the body are determined and controlled by the mind. Kundalini yoga (also known as sahaj, tantra, or siddha yoga) is the path in which the mind is totally surrendered to awakened prana, and the workings of this energy determine the movements of the body. In Kripalu Yoga, the mind is neither totally in control (as in willful practice) nor fully surrendered to the energy (as in Kundalini yoga)—instead, the mind and prana work cooperatively.

Kripalu Yoga is a scientific, workable, experiential system for consciously contacting the usually unconscious workings of the intelligence of prana. It is a revolutionary way of awakening transcendental wisdom at the level of the body, so that it becomes tangible.

Meditation-in-Motion is only possible when the mind works in complete harmony with the body. In fact, Meditation-in-Motion is the expression of body-mind harmony, which becomes the appropriate conduit for the higher intelligence of prana to manifest freely. Thus the first phase of the practice of Kripalu Yoga is essentially dedicated to establishing such body-mind harmony. This becomes the opening for entering the true spirit of yoga. In the final stage of Kripalu Yoga, when the movements of the body are not controlled or guided mentally but prompted directly by the awakened transcendental intelligence of prana, one naturally enters into the experience of transcendental consciousness, even as the body moves.

Because understanding prana as a link between body and mind is the key to successful practice of Kripalu Yoga, this first volume presents a comprehensive explanation of Kripalu Yoga theory. Yogi Desai addresses the entire scope of prana, from its role in the cosmos and creation to its multilevel functioning in the individual human microcosm. Forthcoming volumes will provide detailed instructions for the practice of Kripalu Yoga and present extensive applications.

Yogi Desai has a rare talent for making the previously impenetrable esoteric and abstract teachings about prana approachable, comprehensible, and practical. His own awakening and self-realization are the source of his inspired teachings. The long-term preparation and purification he went through due to his consistent dedicated practice of the willful disciplines of hatha and raja yoga (under the guidance of one of the greatest living Kundalini masters, Swami Shri Kripalvanandji[4]) enabled him to realize the value, depth, and implications of his posture-flow experience. The system he developed from it gives new depth and meaning to the practice of yoga. He emphasizes that the practice of willful disciplines is of great importance because they are foundational but

[4]See p. 107.

he points out that they serve their true purpose only if we ultimately transcend them.

Yogi Desai's language is at once understandable and inspiring. He has remarkably translated his clear explanations into a practical system so wide-reaching that it encompasses not simply yoga but our view of life itself. He reveals that we can enhance our health, vitality, and well-being; discover solutions to a wide range of life's problems; as well as explore our human and divine potential fully—all merely by learning to use the wisdom of this unrecognized intelligence we all possess. Kripalu Yoga then does not just remain confined to its formal practice but becomes a way of life.

Whether you are an experienced yoga practitioner who chooses to expand the scope and benefits of your current practice by incorporating these transforming principles, or someone brand new to yoga, the revelatory material Yogi Desai offers in this book will help you find a new relevance, deep fulfullment, and joy in your practice that can extend throughout every area of your life.

Introduction

Hidden within your body and mind exists the awesome power of the life force that yogis call prana. When awakened, prana can be used as a powerful catalyst to transform your life. It is accessible and available to everyone equally; yet very few have learned the secrets of awakening and using this energy to fulfill their highest human potentials. Most of those who have used this force have discovered it intuitively or accidentally; few have used it consciously. Until now, the knowledge of how to awaken and channel prana has remained a mystery known only to great masters of the world—particularly the yogis of India.

It is my intention in this book to make ancient yogic teachings on prana available to everyone that they can be easily understood, applied in a practical way, and experienced. Anyone can consciously use the higher intelligence of this miraculous force lying dormant within each one of us. Once you learn how to become aware of this energy and how to awaken it, you have an unlimited force working for you from within, providing perpetual inspiration, strength, and courage for realizing your inner growth through any activity you choose.

What I am presenting in this volume is not just philosophy or intellectual theory, but the result of my own direct experience. Attuning to the workings of prana transformed my life and completely changed my perception and practice of yoga. It gave me the facility to enter depths of yoga I never imagined existed and some of the claims of yoga that I had perceived to be reserved for only a chosen few great spiritual masters and saints became real for me.

The Birth of Meditation-in-Motion

In 1970 during my routine practice of hatha yoga postures I found my body moving spontaneously and effortlessly while at the same time I was being drawn into the deepest meditation I had ever experienced. The power and intelligence that guided me through this seemingly paradoxical experience of meditation and motion left me in awe and bliss. That morning my body moved of its own volition, without my direction, automatically performing an elaborate series of flowing motions. Many of these "postures" I had never seen even in any yoga book before. It was the movements of my body—which ordinarily are thought to be an obstruction to concentration—that drew my outgoing attention inward and brought about the inner stillness of deepest meditation. This induced an expanded state of consciousness that revealed new dimensions of life and filled me with ecstasy. Later my joy was even greater when I found I was able to enter the same experience again and again during my daily practice.

Each time I returned to my everyday activities, I returned with this consciousness. I found myself working, perceiving, and interacting from a whole new level of spontaneity, rather than striving for spiritual ideals or acting from habitual behavior and adopted beliefs. Just as my posture flow experience was not mentally contrived, forced, or controlled, when I came out of it all my interactions and activities—whether spiritual disciplines or worldly responsibilities—became more and more spontaneous. The powerful initial impact was progressively deepened by my daily yoga practices.

This started a profound transformation of both my inner and outer life that is still unfolding today, more than fifteen years later. Soon after my experience I learned that what triggered this ongoing process is described in the ancient yogic texts as the activation of my own life force—the awakening of prana.

Miraculous Results

From that day in 1970, my practice became a richly rewarding and deeply joyous experience. The unusual depth I consistently reached in my new practice perpetually revealed to me that this force that manifested through my body was an intelligence greater than my mind could ever comprehend or duplicate, and that it could take care of all my unrecognized internal needs better than I ever could. Through my practice of this Meditation-in-Motion daily the awakened energy worked out tensions and painful strains throughout my body; brought me great vitality, muscle tone, and flexibility; and produced internal healings.

But these were only the more obvious, visible, external workings of this new-found higher intelligence that consistently surprised me. Along with the removal of the tensions at the muscular level, the movements of the body were also cathartic at the mental and emotional levels and would occasionally bring up some forgotten incident, and unresolved feelings from my past would flash through my awareness without any identifiable cause. Each time this happened I felt a release and an unburdening that was experienced as joy. Truly a grace had descended upon me that was working out old karma lodged far beyond the reach of my awareness.

Thus through these releases the energy continually brought about purification at a deeper and deeper level. Seeing its amazing workings over and over again, I developed an enduring trust in this inner source that performed miracles of healing and opened new doors for my spiritual growth by triggering my faith in a force greater than my conscious mind. Until then I had only heard about an "evolutionary urge" and such terms as "higher self," "inner voice," etc. and they were only ideal concepts beyond my grasp. But I had never really known what was now experientially revealed to me as I realized the workings of this higher intelligence through my body.

Once I learned how to let it work freely, this intelligence worked perfectly without my having to know, understand, control, or make it manifest according to my preconceived ideals or plans. Often before, in my pursuit of personal development through the practice of yoga or other activities, there was a subtle striving that created internal struggle and conflict within both my body and mind. Such forced disciplines that were supposed to reduce my internal tensions were on a subtle level actually producing them. All of a sudden, all the striving that happened in the name of my higher growth was not necessary and naturally dropped as the spontaneous working of this higher intelligence took over.

It was the greatest discovery of my life. Yet this most mysterious and powerful healing, rejuvenating, and enlightening force that lies right beneath the surface in everyone, remains unknown to most people throughout their lives. Only after my experience could I see how easily accessible it is.

When Prana Awakens

Prana is the animating force of the entire universe. It functions in our bodies day and night, from birth to death. It carries out all the life-sustaining processes known as our involuntary functions. In what I call its dormant state, this intelligence works at this biological/survival level. As miraculous as it is, this survival-level working is prana's lower-level functioning. When awakened, prana acts on an evolutionary level. At its evolutionary expression, prana functions with the same intelligence and just as automatically as it does at the involuntary level, but at a highly accelerated rate. Awakened prana works not only on a biological level but also works out deep-seated psychological and emotional blocks. As this activated energy awakens higher consciousness, an individual life expresses more universal qualities such as intuition, faith, trust, love, and compassion. The awakening of prana thus opens a whole new dimension of life as well as adding new depth to the formal practice of yoga.

A New Yoga

The awakening of prana is the prior stage of what in the yogic texts is known as Kundalini awakening.

Although over the years before my experience I had read some of the literature on Kundalini yoga and heard of its mysterious workings, it was far beyond my comprehension. At that time, perhaps, I never paid much attention to what was said as I never suspected it could ever happen to me. But after my experience I began to study and research the subjects of Kundalini and prana more extensively. The ancient teachings that formerly seemed obscure and vague became clear in the light of my experience.

The practice of Kundalini yoga, in which one receives the grace and benefits of the activated cosmic intelligence, prana, has been known to the great yogis of India for thousands of years, but it has been kept secret. It became obvious to me that the ancient masters must have intentionally written these powerful teachings in an esoteric language to prevent them from being misused by those who were not ready for Kundalini awakening, which produces cathartic experiences so intense it is beyond the scope of most people who have not totally dedicated their lives to the practice of yoga. To share my experience I wanted to find a way to incorporate and integrate the benefits of prana in the formal practice of yoga and daily life without having to go as far as the awakening of Kundalini.

This led me to years of research and study and experimentation on myself and with many of my students that ultimately enabled me to develop a new approach to the practice of yoga. With this system of practical techniques, anyone can incorporate the remarkable benefits of awakened prana into the traditional practice of hatha yoga and consciously enter into spontaneous Meditation-in-Motion.

I consider this experience to be a special grace of my beloved guru, Swami Shri Kripalvanandji. It is in his honor that I named this new method Kripalu Yoga.

Kripalu Yoga: The Science of Unlearning

Difficulty in the practice of yoga is not so much in learning what we do not know, but in unlearning what we have acquired so that what is inborn may manifest. The true practice of yoga is founded on the principle that we are born with every quality and strength we need already present within. These are popularly known as intuition, insight, inner knowing, the inner voice, inspiration, etc. But these capacities, which are the higher evolutionary manifestation of prana, are nonfunctional or inaccessible when they are suppressed by learned belief systems, concepts, habits and other behavior patterns and attitudes, and preoccupation with meeting goals and ideals.

Therefore the whole practice of Kripalu Yoga is learning how to remove the mental suppressions and inhibitions that keep this higher intelligence from manifesting. Kripalu Yoga is not for acquiring any so-called new knowledge from external sources but to awaken that which is already inborn. It is an ongoing process of removing obstacles at physical, mental, and emotional levels. In the process, every stage of removal you go through releases the life force and helps in regaining health and vitality not only at the level of the body, but also of the mind, which can then turn its attention to our real needs. There is no need to bring in higher knowledge—the removal of the obstruction automatically becomes the process of awakening.

The Zen of Kriaplu Yoga

Thus in Kripalu Yoga, traditional hatha yoga postures are used with a purpose much greater than the way they are used popularly. They become a vehicle for meditative experience as a means to awaken the intelligence of prana and thereby activate higher levels of consciousness. Through their practice we learn how to empty the mind of its acquired attitudes and predispositions that block this energy. In this sense postures play a similar role as the various arts and sports do in zen, such as the practice of archery, judo, the tea ceremony, etc. Just as the purpose of zen archery is not merely to hit the target; the purpose of the martial arts not just to overcome the enemy; and the purpose of koans not to find the answer to a question; so also in Kripalu Yoga the purpose of the practice of asanas is not merely to perfect the postures or derive their physical benefits, but rather to use them as a tool to transcend all physical and mental limitations of the conditioned mind to awaken to our highest potential.

The Joyful Practice

Kripalu Yoga is the yoga of energy, designed so that the wisdom of the body becomes the leading authority that automatically prioritizes its own needs and tailors its movements to fill them. In the absence of having to control movement to conform to any technique or to perfect the posture—in the absence of any such striving to meet any standards or to conform to any authority—the body's movements are so relaxed, so spontaneous, and so effortless, inner creativity begins to manifest without any restrictions, and the mind becomes so enchanted that the experience of yoga becomes deeply satisfying and self-affirming. The working of the energy is so awe-producing, so relaxing, and so fulfilling that practice is no longer a discipline, but instead becomes a joy.

Practical Applications of Prana Theory

No matter in what field you apply Kripalu Yoga principles, you will arrive at a stage of thoughtless, effortless, blissful spontaneity. Whether the expression is of yoga, art, sports, music—or any other activity—it will flow from the unrestricted source of your innermost core of creativity.

In my research and study I found that the principles that help awaken prana have been applied in recent approaches to sports, such as the *Inner Game of Tennis*, *Inner Skiing*, etc., since any capacity we want to expand that goes beyond surface consciousness invariably uses the force of prana. Yet these popular approaches are not geared for awakening but for its preliminary application, using the internal wisdom of the body as a source of playing an effective game and as a method of quick and effective learning. Though Kripalu Yoga principles can also be used for enhanced performance at sports or any other activity, that is not their purpose. Kripalu Yoga emphasizes self-realization.

God Is Energy

What religions have called the grace of God or the workings of the spirit is actually the working of the life force of prana within us. The process of tuning in to prana is a direct way of experiencing this universal higher intelligence. It removes any abstract concepts of "God" as it makes it possible to experience God working in the body. Its blessings come not from any god outside of you, but from freeing the energy of this divine intelligence working through you. Thus Kripalu Yoga becomes a concrete way of experiencing grace, not somewhere in a remote or imagined future, but immediately and palpably. This grace is always present, and when the elements suppressing it are removed, the spirit prana is automatically experienced.

The direct way of experiencing this universal intelligence is through the medium of surrender. My own experience of 1970 was the result of the surrender that emerged naturally when my mind took a back seat and stopped interfering with the free workings of prana: my mind surrendered to the intelligence working through my body. Often, the word "surrender" raises fears because it is interpreted as loss of control. Actually, surrender in this sense means giving over to a wiser, more protective part of yourself that does a better job of caring for you than your conditioned mind can. In other words, your mind is surrendered to your own higher self.

When you begin to see this force that performs miracles in your body with greater intelligence than you can ever achieve, you naturally discover that you are not just your body and your mind. Faith and trust, which ordinarily remain as speculative as the concept of God, emerge naturally, inspired by such a direct personal experience of the workings of this undeniable intelligence. This faith then becomes the foundation for the greater manifestation of this force. Understanding prana as God's intelligence working through us forms the basis of Kripalu Yoga. The very purpose of the practice is to go back to the purity of prana's expression to lift all the individual distortions that ordinarily control and inhibit its working.Prana is divine intelligence alive in our bodies and to harness this energy is to turn the idea of God into an experiential tangible reality, and a force for healing, rejuvenation and accelerated evolution of consciousness.

By presenting in modern terms the relationship of prana to body, mind, breath, emotions, spirit, and to personal transformation and evolution, I hope to give the formerly vague and esoteric, philosophical representation of prana a new relevance and usefulness in our everyday lives as well as in the practice of yoga. I hope the study of the philosophy of Kripalu Yoga helps you to incorporate its principles in your own daily practice to experience the same ecstasy and realization that transformed my life. I wish you great joy in your practice of Kripalu Yoga, and your discovery of prana—the divine intelligence within.

Yogi Amrit Desai
Lenox, Massachusetts

Yogi Amrit Desai

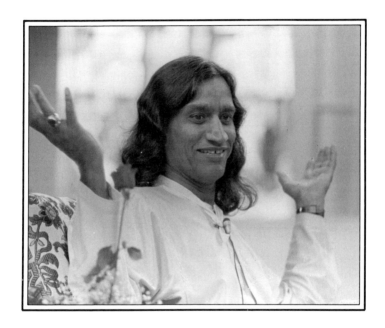

To be with Yogi Amrit Desai (often known as Gurudev) is, for many, an unforgettable experience. His is a strong, joyful, uplifting energy of love and wisdom. He feels like someone very familiar, very near and dear, even from the first encounter. His love, which he extends to each person he meets, has a child-like quality of openness and purity. His unconditional acceptance which is so obvious in both his life and his teachings, inspires love and trust.

Yogi Desai began yoga when he first met his guru, Swami Kripalvanandji in 1948 at the age of 16, but it was a profound spiritual experience in 1970 (described in this book) that transformed his life. Shortly afterwards, he received shaktipat initiation from his guru. Since then the energy awakened within him has had a powerful spiritual influence on the people who come close to him. That event marked the real beginning of his spiritual work, and this led to the development of Kripalu Yoga as well as Kripalu Yoga Ashram in 1970.

Yogi Desai says, "I was fortunate enough to be the disciple of one of the great Masters of India, Swami Kripalvanandji. He practiced Kundalini yoga meditation ten hours a day for the last thirty years of his life. He practiced total silence for twelve years; the last ten years he spoke publicly only twice a year. Through his rigorous sadhana of total dedication to God he reached to the highest stage of *Nirvikalpa Samadhi*. I was specially privileged to be one of his closest disciples, and to receive the most sacred gift of his spiritual heritage. He not only gave me *shaktipat diksha,* but he also empowered me to give shaktipat to sincere seekers to carry on this work in the West."

Yogi Desai is a universal teacher, and freely incorporates into his own teachings those of all masters and religions of the world. His words touch the hearts of people of all nationalities, religions, and walks of life. He is in demand as a speaker all over the world, and is the author of many books translated into several languages. Having been born in India, studied under a great Master, and taught for 25 years in the West, he is able to teach this secret wisdom of the East without losing the depth, quality, and purity of the ancient teachings. He teaches in practical terms that are easy to understand and to incorporate into the modern way of life.

His teachings come from his direct contact with his innermost being and knowing, and as a result are spontaneous, original, and universal. He speaks directly to the very core of our being. He says, "There is nothing I can teach you that you do not already know. All my teaching is but a reminder which your innermost knowing will confirm. In that sense, you already know what I have to say—yet these familiar ingredients combined in a new recipe that is a result of my direct realizations can become a source of new inspiration for you." His discourses have a way of speaking to the deepest questions of the heart, so that at the end each person feels "He was talking directly to me!" Thousands come to him and leave their problems at his feet, healed and refreshed by his presence and counsel.

Yogi Desai is an enlightened Master with penetrating insight and intuition. Whereas most of us may have a moment once in a while where we see to the core of reality, and sense the beauty, harmony, love, and unity behind the apparent diversity and disharmony, he lives in that perpetual awareness. Moreover, he has the ability to raise others to that state of consciousness and teach them how to integrate the experience into their lives so that they, too, can enter into similar levels of awareness. He does not personally claim any of this.

After his transforming experience in 1970, he went into seclusion to deepen his personal spiritual practices, but his loving nature and ability as a teacher attracted many sincere seekers who wanted to learn from him. Thus his sadhana became teaching and sharing with others rather than meditation in solitude. Since then he has dedicated his life to help others grow, and to see that happen is his greatest joy. Swami Kripalvanandji wrote about Yogi Desai: "If someone were to ask me, 'Among your householder disciples[1], whom do you consider most evolved?' I would definitely nominate Amrit first! Amrit is extremely loving; he is fond of sadhana and loves the saints and the scriptures; and he has invoked love for his guru in the hearts of thousands of disciples. His life is like that of a saint."

Yogi Desai has created and directed several ashrams and health centers. The first Ashram was born in 1970. The number of ashram residents grew steadily and to accommodate the growing number of seekers, a larger second Yoga Retreat was acquired in 1975 near Summit Station, Pennsylvania. There, in 1979, Yogi Desai created the Holistic Health Center which has grown into one of the largest and finest of its kind in the country. In 1983, to accommodate growing demands, the present Kripalu Center for Yoga and Health was established in Stockbridge, Massachusetts, which can accommodate 230 staff and nearly 400 guests. It offers a wide range of programs in yoga, holistic health, and personal growth, serving thousands of guests each year. It has 45 branches in North America, Europe, and India.

Yogi Desai has been honored repeatedly by the

---

[1] Yogi Desai has a wife and three children.

spiritual leaders of India and by the American academic community for his mastery of yoga, for his remarkable accomplishments as a spiritual teacher, and for his service to humanity. His Holiness Jagadguru Shankaracharya, one of the foremost spiritual authorities in India, conferred on him an honorary Doctor of Yogic Science degree (1974) in appreciation of his outstanding contributions to humanity and his knowledge of yoga. He was also awarded the title Acharya Pravaraha (Supreme Spiritual Teacher) (1975) by Swami Vedavyasanandji, Chancellor of Rishikul Sanskrit University in Haridwar, India. The title Yogacharya (Spiritual Preceptor) (1980) was conferred by His Holiness Swami Shri Kripalvanandji in honor of his mastery in teaching the spiritual principles and the practices of yoga. He was also given the title Maharishi (Great Sage) (1982) by his Holiness Swami Shri Gangeshwaranandji Udasin, 102 year-old spiritual preceptor, who is highly revered throughout India. In spite of these and other titles, he typically prefers to be called simply Gurudev or Yogi Desai.

Yogi Desai once said:

*"I have not come to teach you,
but to love you;
love itself will teach you."*

His life and works affirm these words.

Chapter One:
The Discovery
of Kripalu Yoga

My First Experience of the
Spontaneous Posture Flow

One morning in 1970 I was performing my daily routine of yoga postures in the meditation room of my home in Philadelphia. With me were my wife, Urmila, and two of my students, John and his wife, Barbara. As was our daily custom, we were all greeting the dawn with stretching, postures and breathing exercises. As an experienced hatha yoga teacher who had practiced yoga for more than twenty years, I could assume the various positions almost effortlessly.

A tape recording of yogic chanting by my guru, Swami Shri Kripalvanandji, played in the background. The intonations of his voice and the gentle background accompaniment of the drum stirred feelings of love and deep reverence within me that led me to perform my daily routine with special concentration that morning. As I continued to move, I became absorbed in the rhythm of the chants. Gradually I became more and more relaxed and absorbed, even while my body continued to move. My movements flowed with the chanting.

The Ecstasy of Inner Awakening

Suddenly, like an unexpected spring downpour, bliss flooded throughout my entire being, and I felt myself being irresistibly drawn to another level of consciousness. As my mind was drawn more and more inward, and the external surroundings dissolved far into the background, I began to feel that I was no longer the performer of the exercises; they were being performed through me.

A new flow of energy coursed throughout my system, and with no conscious effort on my part, my body spontaneously began to twist and turn on its own, flowing smoothly from one posture to the next. The movements were effortless and free, a command and a gift from a newly opened, higher dimension of my inner being. My body became extraordinarily elastic and stretched smoothly and easily beyond its previous limits. I was moving in perfect rhythm with the whole universe. I was not aware of giving any direction to the movements.

Thoughts continued to come, but now they passed through my mind in slow motion, seemingly disconnected from my body's activity. I realized that if I wished, I could stop this experience, and yet I had no desire to do so. Normally, I would decide what posture we would do, and then I would lead the group into it. Although my eyes were closed, I became distinctly aware that the others in the room had silently stopped their own exercises to watch me. I felt some concern for my wife, who might become alarmed by this mysterious state which had overtaken me, but my experience was so profoundly beautiful that I was unwilling to stop the movements of my body.

One after another the postures flowed. Some of them were traditional yoga exercises; others were movements which I had never seen before. Gradually, I became more and more absorbed in my experience. At the end of this flow of postures, my body naturally entered the lotus position, and a deep stillness, so deep that it penetrated every level of my being. Then a second explosion of ecstasy spread through me, and I became engulfed, overwhelmed, by a state of complete inner bliss.

My consciousness slowly began to return to normal. With considerable effort, I was able to open my eyes, discovering to my amazement that it was about thirty minutes later and I was still in my own home surrounded by Urmila, Barbara, and John.

My perceptions of colors, sound, light, and touch were sharper, keener, and clearer. My mind was so clear and my body so completely relaxed that sights and sounds became pure and vibrant. Colors were more lively, with subtler hues than usual. I experienced sounds as if I were dissolving and merging into them. I felt an intimate awareness of life pulsating through everything. I felt at one with everything. The only way I can now describe the feeling is to say that I felt as though I had emerged into a totally new world of harmony, balance, and peace. It was difficult to move, and my breath was almost imperceptible. My face was completely devoid of expression, deeply relaxed and immobile. My mouth was dry, and I realized that I had not swallowed for a long time. I tried to speak, but words would not form.

My friends mirrored my meditative state. As I looked at their unmoving, perfectly peaceful eyes, it seemed that they, too, had entered a deep state of meditation without closing their eyes, and that my experience had communicated itself to them without my saying a word. Gradually and with great difficulty, they began to describe what they had observed while watching me. As they slowly and quietly expressed their experience, I was amazed to hear each of them report a profound, compelling, meditative experience. We struggled to find words to capture this unusual event. From their facial expressions, tone of voice, feelings, and words it was apparent to me that their experience had been similar to my own.

Barbara spoke first. Her eyes maintained the steady, calm gaze of someone who had just come out of deep meditation. In a soft, almost inaudible voice, she broke the deep silence and whispered, "I felt as if I were doing the postures with you."

The others slowly nodded confirmation. They, too, had experienced it. John spoke slowly: "I felt some new force take you over and begin to move your body. A brilliant light surrounded you. It was a completely new experience for me. I've never seen lights or any such phenomena before."

Barbara and Urmila were astonished. Each of them had seen a similar bright glow during the postures. Impressed by the consistency of their experiences, I asked Urmila for her comments. Moved with deep emotion, my wife said, "It didn't seem as if you were doing the postures. They looked so effortless, as

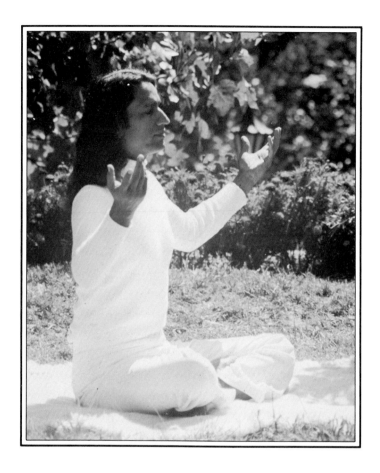

if they were done without your control. They seemed almost—automatic."

The Secrets of My Experience Revealed

Automatic! The word rang with sharp clarity in my mind, evoking the long-forgotten memory of an incident which occurred in India in 1950. I was a young boy of 17, full of enthusiasm for yoga. Swami

Kripalvanandji, whom I called Bapuji[1], had just accepted me as his disciple, and every day before and after school I would desert my schoolbooks and rush to be with him at Gau Mandir, a small, secluded building on the outskirts of my home town[2] where he did his sadhana of Kundalini meditation regularly ten hours a day. One day towards late afternoon I was demonstrating yoga postures, which I learned from a wall poster in a local gymnasium, to some younger school friends on the ground floor beneath Bapuji's meditation room when he happened to come down the stairs. Unnoticed by me, he stopped, so that I would not be disturbed, and silently observed my entire demonstration.

The next day, in order to inspire me, Bapuji granted me a privilege I learned later he has never given anyone else: to be present in his meditation room for a short time while he was in his Kundalini yoga meditation. Very eager to be with him, I hurried to Gau Mandir. Bapuji received me graciously, and closed the door. He proceeded to enter into a deep meditative state. I watched in amazement as his body began to display a remarkable flow of yogic postures, *mudras*[3], and dance-like movements, gracefully and effortlessly flowing from one posture to the next with varying speed and rhythm. After a few minutes

---

[1] An informal but respectful title used by disciples for Swami Shri Kripalvanandji. "Bapu" means "dear father" in Sanskrit, and "-ji" is a respectful suffix.

[2] Halol, in Gujarat State, India.

[3] Mudras are automatic dance-like hand movements.

Bapuji concluded his practices. Then he explained, "My son, all of these innumerable postures, movements, and mudras that you saw me perform occur automatically when the evolutionary energy of prana has been awakened in the body of a yogi. Yogis call this awakening of prana 'pranotthana'. This is an integral part of the awakening of Kundalini."

Bapuji's explanation was completely beyond the comprehension of my young mind. I had always done yoga postures deliberately with conscious control, so I was at a loss to conceive how such movements could occur automatically. But because my respect and love for Bapuji were so great, I did not disbelieve him either. I accepted the fact that some things were beyond my experience, but I did not reject that which I could not grasp at the time. Within a short time, I forgot the event.

Now, twenty years later, Urmila's comment "automatic" brought back the memory of that incident. Was my experience similar to Bapuji's that I had witnessed in his meditation room? Was it the result of the awakened life energy, prana, within me? This was hard for me to believe, because even though I knew very little about the awakening of prana, I had always assumed that a flow of automatic body movements implied an absence of all thought. Yet, thoughts had occurred intermittently during the early part of my experience. Thus, I concluded that my experience could not have been the same flow of automatic postures. And yet, what was the explanation? Intrigued and eager to clarify what had happened to me, I wrote to Bapuji for his interpretation and guidance. In the meantime I found to my delight that I was able to repeat the same experience day after day in my morning postures.

Shortly afterwards I received from Bapuji a typically precise and thorough reply to my questions. Bapuji wrote:

> My son, your experience was indeed the result of the awakening of your life energy, prana. This awakening can happen by the grace of God, guru, or through the study and practice of the disciplines as given in the yogic scriptures. As a result of the awakening of the prana, the body spontaneously begins to perform postures, breathing exercises, and other necessary movements (*kriyas*). These kriyas purify the body and mind. During your visit to India last year, I gave you mild *shaktipat*[1] and special *sadhana*[2] to awaken this energy. Even though these practices which I gave you, along with shaktipat, were meant to awaken prana, I withheld their purpose from you. Due to your appropriate practice of these techniques, you have been fortunate to receive the benediction of the awakening of prana, known as pranotthana.

---

[1] In shaktipat initiation the evolutionary life energy of prana is awakened in the disciple by the grace of the guru.

[2] Sadhana is spiritual practices.

My Body's Inner Wisdom

This experience turned out to be a transforming spiritual event and a turning point in my own life. I had always enjoyed the willful practice of hatha yoga postures very much, but now my sadhana took on a totally new twist. I fell in love with yoga practices as I never had before. I found that each time my mind was totally engaged in the experience; I remained awe-struck and absorbed. My postures were no longer a discipline but a sheer joy as my body became deeply relaxed and extremely limber. Every day I entered into deep meditative experiences while my body was guided into various positions. My mind felt as if it melted into the rush of energy, into the sensations and feelings that emerged from the depths of my being. My yoga practice became a flowing uncensored music of the soul that felt more like a prayer than practice of postures. Each time I was transported into pure inner bliss I transcended all sense of space and time. I felt as though I was entering into a sacred experience, into the eternal Now. My body seemed to become ever more alive and sensitive.

As my body's inner wisdom took over and directed my movements, my mind, with its traditional learned ways of doing yoga practice, rested in the background, watching in great amazement. My movements, postures, resting periods, and breath patterns were all choreographed and synchronized with great intelligence, superior to any that I had ever known through my conscious mind during my previous daily practice of yoga. In spite of all the knowledge of yoga that I had acquired over a long period of study, I had never been able to tune in to my own individual needs with such precision. I had practiced a fixed routine, a traditional approach to hatha yoga and hardly paid any attention to my body's needs. This intelligence of prana knew what to do, how long to hold a posture, and what the next movement would be. All choices of movement and postures originated from somewhere deep within my body and were precisely designed to meet my individual needs on any given day at any given time. There was no set sequence. Each day my body's internal needs chose new combinations of postures. The familiar routine and traditional way of practice became secondary and the inner wisdom of the body that came in the form of urges that guided and choreographed the movements became primary. This made my daily practice a refreshing experience, a new and constant source of joy for me.

I also had repeated experiences of the healing wisdom of prana during times of physical pain. Every time, I found that if I just relaxed totally and allowed prana to move my body in spontaneous postures, this inner intelligence would know exactly what movements to make to get rid of the pain almost instantly. Often these movements were almost imperceptible — I have called them "micromovements." Often, too, they were not at the location of the pain but were in an apparently unrelated part of the body.

Before my experiences with prana, when I had similar problems, I would try to consciously adjust my body at the site of the pain in the way that I *thought* would or should relieve the tension. I would sometimes end up irritating the injury and making it worse!

In this new way, pain that would normally have stayed with me for days or even weeks, was gone by the end of my session of moving meditation. I was also able to guide others into similar experiences.

This is just a simple, understandable example of how prana's healing wisdom is superior to that of the habitual thinking mind or any external authority. I have seen many such profound and apparently miraculous healings from prana's workings. To tune into this wisdom, faith and trust in the natural process are necessary because they are conducive to relaxation, which is what activates prana. So-called faith healing is actually the workings of prana freed up as a result of deep relaxation.

Before this, I had always trusted the information from books, ancient traditions or other external authorities far more than I trusted my own body both in yoga and health and diet. Now I see that all such information is secondhand and generalized, whereas my body's wisdom is tailored personally and specifically to my need at any given time. So now I go back to the first and only book, the source of all scriptures, the wisdom of prana expressed through the body.

How Could I Share this Ecstatic Experience?

In all my twenty-two years of formal yoga practice, I had never entered such deep and blissful states of consciousness even in my meditations, let alone

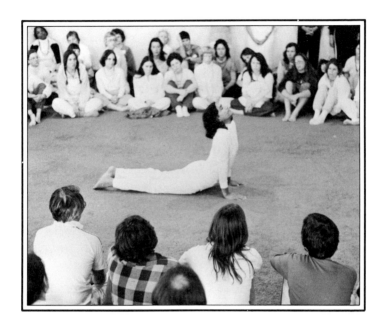

during my traditional hatha yoga practice. My great desire was now to find a way to share this ecstatic experience with others. As I entered daily into the spontaneous meditative posture flow, I realized that my ability to recreate the appropriate conditions again and again was intuitive rather than consciously planned. I also realized that this intuitive ability was the result of my many years practice and study of willful yoga.

I began to observe my new experience in light of my previous yoga practices to make conscious the conditions that had created it, so as to be able to formalize them into an approach that would give others an opportunity to have the experience of spontaneous postures that had revealed to me the true depths of yoga. After I had read the letter of my guru and realized that my experience was due to the awakening of prana, I had decided to study the ancient science of *prana vidya*[1], the science of freeing and awakening prana and Kundalini, known to yogis for thousands of years.

I had always known that Bapuji practiced Kundalini sadhana many hours a day, but I had never studied the subject of prana or Kundalini awakening in depth before because it had no relevance to my own practice. My sadhana was different—I was living a householder's life and practicing hatha yoga in the traditional way (Kundalini yoga is generally practiced in seclusion). I never suspected that one day I would experience prana awakening.

My understanding of prana gradually increased as each day I both studied ancient scriptures and also continued to observe the workings of this mysterious inner intelligence during my daily experiences of what I later came to call *"Meditation-in-Motion."*

Prana and Shaktipat

A short time later, I received another letter from Bapuji. In it he wrote:

> My dear son, Amrit: In ancient times a guru gave shaktipat initiation to a deserving disciple of a high moral caliber who was not attached to worldly temptations. After re-

---

[1] Prana vidya is the ancient science of the mastery of prana. There are many systems and approaches to this science, often under the same name.

ceiving shaktipat initiation, the disciple does not need to strive for knowledge, as all the necessary knowledge, guidance, and protection flows from the awakened prana. The disciple, however, has to one-pointedly dedicate his life to spiritual practices. It is my wish that you be prepared to give shaktipat to your deserving students, so that your virtuous, blessed mission of spreading the teachings of yoga in the West may be well-fulfilled. When you return to India again in January, I will seat you in front of me and bestow upon you the yogic power to give shaktipat to your students so that the sacred tradition of imparting shaktipat initiation will be protected and perpetuated.

Shaktipat: The Answer?

After three months of intensive practices and study with my guru, I formally received shaktipat initation from him, along with the rare blessing of the ability to give shaktipat initiation to others.

At first this seemed to be the answer to my intense desire to share my blissful experience with others. For a while I closely observed all those who experienced prana awakening through contact with me, and who had many ecstatic meditative experiences of spontaneous postures and other involuntary movements.[1] However, those people consistently ex-

---

[1] Butler, 1979 (see Bibliography).

posed to prana shakti (energy) also experienced so much intense emotional catharsis and physical purification that it affected their ability to carry out their normal daily responsibilities. They were often moody and irritable, and also found that their sexual energy became overactive.

Need for a Firm Foundation of Willful Practice

Therefore I discontinued giving shaktipat, realizing that such prana awakening, which in fact is an early stage of Kundalini awakening, was premature for them. I saw it was important for students to first lay a firm foundation for physical purification through willful yoga practices and also to purify the mind of desires, attachments and fears, both of which Bapuji had directed me to do for many years prior to my prana awakening. Without such a foundation, the catharsis stimulated by awakened prana was too difficult to digest and process constructively. I realized that these students would also have to make radical changes in their lifestyle in order to support the inner workings of awakened energy, and that they were not yet ready for that. This realization led me to begin to develop a new, step-by-step method of willful yoga practices and appropriate lifestyle guidelines which would progressively prepare the students for a more gradual awakening of prana. This was the beginning of Kripalu Yoga.

Prana: The Ultimate Fulfillment of Yoga Practice

Because all yogic disciplines have been specifically designed to eventually awaken prana, we definitely benefit a great deal from practicing them willfully even without knowing the secrets of prana. But from my own personal experience I knew consciously allowing prana to work more freely in the body gives a totally new dimension to the usual willful practice of postures.

It is possible to enjoy the benefits of yoga without prana awakening, but it tends to become mechanical, uninteresting, and even boring at times. Such lack of interest misses the very spirit of yoga. This spirit is what I had rediscovered through prana awakening, and I wanted to infuse it into regular willful practice, so that the true depth of yoga would be experienced even at an early stage.

In the process of developing Kripalu Yoga it became clear to me that many of the benefits of freed-up prana can indeed be incorporated into willful practices, even without the actual awakening of prana itself. So even the earlier stages of the five-stage Kripalu Yoga technique make use of this principle of prana vidya, the freeing[1] and awakening of prana. Through Kripalu Yoga the student learns experientially about the laws of prana and its relationship to body, mind, breath and spirit. Applying this knowledge so as to conserve prana and use it wisely, both in formal yoga practices and daily life, provides a tool for the *gradual* acceleration of the body's healing and purification processes, which formerly was available only through sudden, intense prana awakening such as in Kundalini yoga.

Thus, even the willful stages of Kripalu Yoga, as described at the end of this book, are different from the usual willful practice of hatha yoga, because from the start the new depth and dimension of prana is incorporated into daily practice.[2]

This incorporation of the prana principle into hatha yoga postures also lays a firm foundation for the accelerated awakening of prana in the final stage of Kripalu Yoga. This, in turn, is a preparation for awakening prana to greater intensity in Kundalini yoga for those who wish to continue that path.

---

[1] "Freeing Prana" is what I have called the first level of accelerated activity of prana, which is achieved by the preparatory willful stages of Kripalu Yoga. The second level I have called "Prana Awakening", which is achieved in Stage Five of Kripalu Yoga. Kundalini awakening is the awakening of prana to the most accelerated level which carries out purification with the highest intensity. Each of these levels of awakening represents an increase in the cathartic and evolutionary activity of prana.

[2] Specific techniques for incorporating this principle into daily hatha yoga will be given in the next volume of this series.

Chapter Two:
Prana: The Connecting Link Between Man and the Universe

How Does Prana Work in the Individual and in the Universe?

I continued to expand my theoretical basis for understanding of this complex and fascinating phenomenon of awakened prana (shakti). In addition to my research into prana vidya I began to read Samkhya yoga philosophy and also to study Kundalini yoga in more depth in Bapuji's books, such as **Science of Meditation** and **Asana and Mudra.**[1] These contain not just abstract philosophy but his own deeply experiential wisdom coming from a sadhana of ten hours a day of Kundalini meditation for the last thirty years of his life.

I wanted to learn specifically: *How* does this energy know what to do? *How* does it understand, prioritize, and provide for my inner needs, needs that even I, with all my knowledge of yoga and my great sensitivity to my health and to my body, could not figure out precisely? I started inquiring more in depth:

---

[1] See Bibliography.

- What is prana?
- How is it awakened?
- How can prana move my body, independent of my conscious mind?
- How can I help others to experience it too?
- Can anyone awaken prana without shaktipat from a guru? And if so, how?
- How is my experience of awakening of prana related to the theoretical descriptions of prana as given in the ancient texts?
- What is the relationship of prana to body, mind, breath, and spirit?
- How can prana be awakened at a level of lesser intensity than in Kundalini awakening?

I knew that when I could formulate workable, practical answers to these questions, I would be able to complete the development of a technique which would systematically prepare others for the prana experience that only *appeared* to have happened spontaneously to me, but for which I, too, had been unknowingly prepared through many years of willful practices.

During this formative and experimental period of Kripalu Yoga, I was also in the fortunate position of being able to test my theories and methods on the many hundreds of yoga students and teachers that I was training at that time. From my many years of teaching experience and my in-depth study of prana, I gained many new insights into the secrets of this intelligent energy, which revealed the answers to

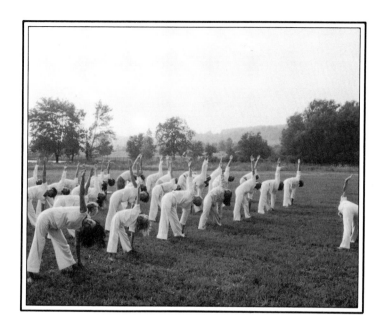

these questions and provided a firm foundation for their practical application in Kripalu Yoga.

Prana: The Source of All That Exists

From Samkhya yoga philosophy and my other readings, I gained an understanding of prana as the intelligent life principle of all that exists, the Prime Cause of the entire creation. This primal life force is the essence of everything that manifests; it regulates the law and order, rhythm and harmony of the entire universe. Prana pervades and interpenetrates all that has been created throughout the cosmos, whether visible or invisible, known or unknown, subtle or gross. It is prana which steers the course of the galaxies, stars, planets, earth, sun, and moon with computer-like precision. Everything in the universe comes into being through prana, is sustained through prana, evolves through prana, and is again dissolved and transformed by prana. This universal life energy is the intelligent evolutionary energy from which every form that is contained within space and time has come into being. Prana is the universal Spirit, unborn, undying, unchanging, and indestructible. It is alpha and omega, without beginning, without end.

Prana Maintains Ecological Balance

This intelligence that guides and regulates the course of galaxies, stars, and planets with utmost precision is the same intelligent energy that regulates the ecological balance and evolution of mineral, plant, animal and human life on the planet Earth. These evolutionary cycles of birth, growth, death, and rebirth are all caused and carried out by the intelligent workings of the creative impulse of prana, the universal soul—God.

Prana's intelligent workings manifest as many different energies throughout our universe, for example: electrical, nuclear, magnetic, and gravitational energies. These forces all work according to precise laws, which we have discovered and formulated through the various physical sciences: physics, chemistry, biology, astronomy, and so on. All these sciences study the manifestations of prana as other energies in the universe at a material level that we can perceive and manipulate. The spiritual sciences study the subtle laws of prana itself that govern our human processes of evolution and growth.

The yogic scriptures make it clear that the miraculously intricate workings of human and animal bodies are sustained by the very same intelligent energy of prana that created and maintains the galaxies and heavenly bodies in space. The same organized and orderly intelligence is responsible for regulating both the ecological balance of life on the planet Earth and the homeostatic balance of human life processes. Thus prana is the cause of the order and precision of both the macrocosm of the universe and the microcosm of the human body.

Prana: Different Names in Different Cultures

I came to realize that this primal energy that yogis call "prana" is the same energy that has been recognized, studied, and even worshipped by many religions, cultures, and civilizations. Mankind has given this energy many names: Holy Spirit, Chi, Cosmic Mind, Bio-energy, Soul, Shakti, Orgone, and Élan Vital, to name but a few. This energy is further explained in Samkhya yoga philosophy as not only the undifferentiated Cosmic Spirit, God, or (in Sanskrit) *Purusha*, the one source of the entire creation, but also as what we recognize manifesting as the individual spirit, the spark of the divine within us. It is through this Spirit that our physical body comes alive. The manifest form or Cosmic Body of unmanifest Purusha is called *Prakriti*. This is how the Creative Spirit comes to us and reveals itself to us through its creation. Purusha, the Cosmic Spirit, and Prakriti, matter, are wedded inseparably together in every expression of the entire creation. So prana exists within each of us as individual spirit, the seed of God. This gives us the potential to realize our inborn oneness with God. As I compared my own experience with what I read of the theoretical teachings about prana, I realized with great joy that the ancient teachings of yoga had come to life in me! At last, I could bridge the gap between the abstract philosophical teachings about prana and the actual experience of awakened prana. I was able to realize experientially my direct connection with this divine energy.[1] Prana now took on a new and deeper meaning and became an integral part of my life and daily practice.

My experience showed me that we can all invoke this divine energy in the temple of our body—that this is not just a poetic allegory but a very real experience. When prana is awakened it is the divine energy of the Cosmic Spirit manifesting in the body. It is a sacred experience, a prayerful communion with the divine such as when I experienced the awakening of prana. What had formerly been merely an abstract theoretical belief in God became an experiential reality for me, so I know that through the practice of prana awakening we can all experience God in this direct way. My whole purpose in developing Kripalu Yoga has been to provide a step-by-step method for

---

[1] Often the awakening of prana is also referred to as the awakening of Divine Mother Kundalini Shakti.

gradually awakening prana, so that anyone who practices consistently and is open and ready can experience this intelligent energy flowing through the body.

The Various Meanings of "Prana"

In the traditional yogic texts, the term "prana" is used to describe several different levels of manifestation and functioning of the life force.[1] I would like to simplify and clarify this overlapping of meanings for the purposes of this volume, and refer to either "Prana" or "prana". I will use "Prana" to refer to the Cosmic Spirit that I described as being the core of the creation, sustenance, and evolution of the entire universe. I will use "prana" (small "p") to refer to the biological energy which animates and sustains all the involuntary life-giving functions within the body. This intelligent working of prana, which I call the wisdom of the body, is a reflection of the intelligence of the universal Spirit, Prana. "Prana" is also traditionally used to refer to the breath (as in pranayama), because the life of the individual begins with the first breath in and ends with the last breath out, and is sustained by a series of uninterrupted breaths in-between. In many cultures breath is conceived of as the spirit.[2] The Hebrew word for "breath of life" can also be translated "spirit of life", as can the Latin "Spiritus." Breath and spirit are thus intimately re-

---

[1] **Devatma Shakti,** pp. 54-69.

[2] *"The Lord God formed man of dust from the ground, and breathed into his nostrils the breath of life, and man became a living soul."* Genesis 2:7.

lated. The interchangeability of these two uses of the word "prana" represents this intimate relationship that exists between breath and prana. Biological energy becomes activated with the first breath, which acts like a flywheel and sets all other life-giving involuntary functions into motion. This intelligent biological energy is also known as *prana-vayu* in the scriptures, but it is often simply referred to as prana.

It is the presence of Spirit, Prana, that enables the body to absorb biological prana from the breath. So you can see that just as breath is the life of the body, Prana, the Spirit, is the life of the life-giving breath. When the Spirit leaves the body, the body can no longer absorb prana from the air. Breath is the carrier of the universal intelligence, Cosmic Spirit, that supports the involuntary intelligence of biological energy, prana-vayu, in our body because of the presence of prana, the individual spirit.

Even though most of us have known only the mind as a source of knowledge and wisdom, obviously there is within us another source of intelligence that is higher than the mind—the wisdom of prana. This source of wisdom resides within each of us, whether we are aware of it or not, and we use it daily; yet its operation within the body has neither been explored nor scientifically studied.

The whole aim and thrust of Kripalu Yoga is to enable us to use this intelligent life energy of prana more consciously for our own healing, personal growth, and spiritual evolution.

Chapter Three:
Prana's Role in Body, Mind, and Evolution

The intelligent energy of prana works like a subtle electricity that travels through the network of our subtle nerves (*nadis*) and nerve centers (*chakras*). This prana-vayu provides the life impulse to all the vital functions within our body.

Prana working at this biological level, which I call the survival or sustenance level, carries out three different types of activities in our body: voluntary, involuntary, and instinctual. The life processes of the autonomic nervous system we have discussed such as respiration, digestion, circulation, and rejuvenation, operate independently of our mind. The instinctual survival urges manifest as fear of heights, fight-or-flight response, etc.. The more voluntary functions include eating, eliminating, procreation, and sleeping. Prana communicates these needs to the mind in the form of bodily messages such as thirst, hunger, fatigue, the urge for elimination, work, rest, sex, and so forth. To provide for the body's needs, the mind must remain attentive to prana and cooperate with prana's signals. Thus, the mind must consciously support the *involuntary* functions of the body with the appropriate *voluntary* actions by practicing the healthy way of life. This provides us with a continual supply of prana to

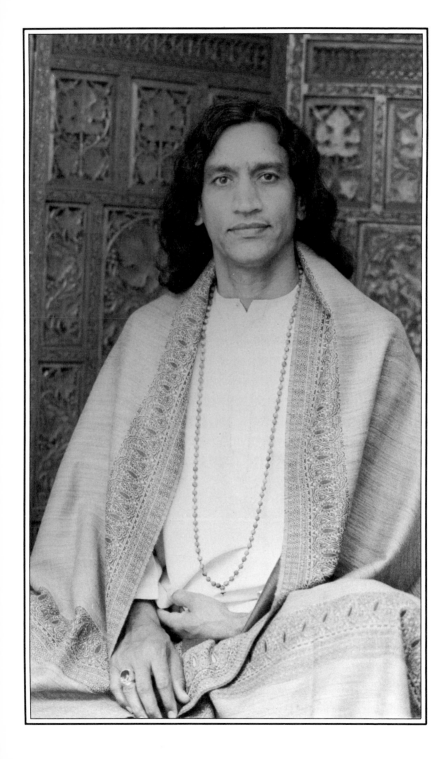

maintain the homeostatic balance of the body, which gives us health and inner harmony.

We need to continually replenish this working energy of prana, as it gets used up both by our involuntary bodily functions and also by our physical, mental and emotional activities and expressions in daily life. As prana is expended in these ways, the homeostatic balance in the body must be continually re-established by taking in more prana. So just as we constantly draw prana for our survival from outside of us through the medium of air, water, food, and sunshine, so also we regain prana and rejuvenate our system during sleep, when we withdraw fully from all external activities. The prana so gained is stored primarily in the solar plexus area, from where it is distributed to other nerve centers and converted into the biological, mental, and emotional energies which we constantly expend in our daily life activities.

Pain: Messenger of Body to Mind

These instinctual and "survival" messages of prana are communicated to the conscious mind with different degrees of intensity. When messages such as need for rest, sleep, and food need to be fulfilled and have been ignored or over-indulged, they will be communicated to us with greater intensity as tension and pain. If they are consistently ignored or over-indulged, eventually they will manifest as chronic and continuous pain and stress, resulting in illness. So prana intensifies its messages to the mind through increased levels of pain until the body's survival needs are met. Thus pain is not there to punish us, but is the way our survival instinct attracts our attention from other preoccupations. We become less sensitive to bodily messages when we are preoccupied by our desires and fears, so more intense messages and severe signals are required for prana to be able to attract our attention. Because our habitual tensions have blocked out these health-giving messages of prana, I have developed the first stage of Kripalu Yoga to begin to dissolve the physical tension blocks so that our mind can respond to the body's needs for survival and sustenance. The freeing of prana is directly related to concentration of mind and deep relaxation of the body. That is why these two play a crucial role in the early stages of Kripalu Yoga.

Necessity for Prana-Mind Cooperation

So, we have two sources of intelligence at our disposal: 1) the limited intelligence of the mind, and 2) the universal intelligence of prana working through the body. It is the responsibility of the mind to attune itself to the needs of the body as signaled by natural bodily urges and to draw upon the external world to provide whatever the body's intelligence requests for sustenance and survival. Thus, the mind's role is to feed and clothe the body, see that it receives proper rest, exercise, play, and see that it eliminates properly. This helps the body to recuperate from the wear and tear that occurs in the natural course of living and to replenish its energy. When mind responds appropriately to the body's needs for energy to carry out both internal involuntary activities and external voluntary activities, mind is in harmony with the body. When the mind supplies the body's needs for food, water, sunshine, play, work, rest, sleep, and elimination, the homeostatic processes within the body are well-maintained and health and vigor are regained daily. This cooperative functioning of the mind and body allows the body's inner intelligence, the involuntary system, to function smoothly and efficiently at the basic, healthy level I call "natural" level. Nature ensures that our survival needs are met by providing us with instinctual urges; these instinctual drives are another level of manifestation of prana's intelligence. In Kripalu Yoga, students learn to attune the mind to these bodily urges so that they can then apply this sensitivity to many other facets of life in order to heal the chronic body-mind breakdown so prevalent in our time.

Prana's Highest Potential: The Evolutionary Urge

In addition to these instinctual and survival urges there is an innate evolutionary urge within us which continually presses for our recognition and inspires us to realize our inborn divine potential. As we take care of the sustenance needs of the body, prana gradually awakens its latent power from this basic "survival" level to an evolutionary level.[1] Thus as we take care of our natural sustenance needs we prepare to

---

[1] This is congruent with Maslow's hierarchy of needs.

move towards our higher human potential. The evolutionary urge exists at a deeper level than the survival instincts and therefore can only be felt when all our survival needs have been satisfied. For example, when our life is in real danger, we put aside all thoughts, ideas, and activities of exploring our higher evolutionary potentials. If your house is on fire you will not be able to meditate. This urge is much gentler, subtler than the more aggressive survival instincts. The purpose of Kripalu Yoga is to become more sensitive so that we uncover this hidden potential, this urge to expand, which is given to all human beings at birth, yet which can remain latent all our lives if we do not become sensitive and consciously awaken it.

When body-mind harmony is achieved through the practice of hatha and raja yogas, which are combined in Kripalu Yoga, then the spiritual seeker can move to higher levels of unfoldment of prana's evolutionary impulse which reveals the divine potentials hidden within us. This occurs because body-mind harmony allows greater attunement to Spirit-Prana's evolutionary impulse within us.

How Mind Can Be an Obstruction to Evolution

Up to and including the level of animal life, evolution on earth happens directly and automatically through the operation of the universal laws of prana, which operate in a uniform way. Animals have no freedom to modify their instinctual or involuntary functions, and so they have no freedom to alter or intervene in the natural evolutionary rhythms. Their lives are sustained by the universal wisdom of prana working through them directly as survival instinct.[1] Animals' life activities of eating, resting, playing, recreation, and procreation happen through instinct; they have no choice but to function in direct harmony with natural laws of health and well-being of the body.

Only we humans, with our unique attribute of choice, given by the higher evolutionary manifestation of prana as mind and consciousness, are an exception to the uniform evolutionary law. We alone can alter our evolutionary rhythm and heighten it to attain the state of ultimate freedom. We as humans have the inborn potential to awaken to higher levels of consciousness beyond the level of instinctive functioning. This gift of mind and consciousness also opens to us the choice to go against the natural laws, so our potential asset is also a potential liability.

When we go against the natural laws of health and harmony it brings misery and pain. The same mind, when tuned into the natural laws which manifest as the intelligence of prana, brings us good health, great joy and happiness in our life, and helps actualize our divine potential.

When body and mind work in harmony, by mind supporting body's needs, this awakens the higher consciousness, which supports the evolutionary urge at all times. When mind ignores the needs of the body,

---

[1] Children function in much the same way, directly from prana, without the intervention of mind, until the individuality begins to manifest.

this potential evolutionary energy is consumed in psychological and physiological tension blocks which result in feelings of self-doubt, fear, and insecurity. When the energy thus entangled in body-mind conflict is released, it is freed to work as higher consciousness. This harmonious working of body and mind to support evolutionary prana is what I have called primal awareness, or "prana-mind." Whenever mind is in conflict with the instinctual urges that support the survival of the body, and the evolutionary urges that support our spiritual potential, I call that "ego-mind."

So mind is the key to our evolution, by either going against our inborn urges or letting us live in tune with them. Mind itself is neutral; it is neither negative nor positive in and of itself. It is like a ladder with which we can choose to go to an upper or a lower level.

How Prana is Used or Abused

Our mind has developed its own separate agenda of unnatural priorities that have nothing to do with the body's real needs. These mental priorities have been artificially and unconsciously acquired through social, cultural, and religious patterns of thinking called "conditioning." Added to these social conditionings and beliefs are many individual habits, fears, and insecurities. Attitudes derived from our unconscious conditioning may lead us into courses of action that are not in accord with prana's wisdom, which represents the universal laws of health, harmony, and evolution. This individual conditioning that is in conflict with the universal wisdom of prana is what I call ego-mind.

Ego-mind is always a victim of habits, intoxicated with the ego's demands for more security through more money, more control, more recognition, and with an insatiable appetite for more pleasure, fun, and excitement. The search to fulfill these desires is so blinding that ego-mind causes us to act against the wisdom of the body. It uses the body as a slave to provide more fun and more pleasure. This makes the body expend its already diminishing bio-energy of prana. Through overuse and constant stress, the body accumulates chronic tensions which reduce its ability to draw prana from food and from breath. Its ability to eliminate waste-products and toxins from the body is also diminished and unhealthy conditions begin to develop. When this happens the involuntary functions of the digestive and eliminative organs are impaired, the homeostatic processes are disturbed, and aging is accelerated. This is how the conditioned mind, cluttered with misleading and self-destructive value systems, leads us into activities that disrupt the normally harmonious workings of prana in our body, and leads us away from higher evolution.

The instinctive "wisdom of the body," prana, is not subject to any such conditioning, so the purpose of Kripalu Yoga is to bypass all the conditionings of the mind by learning to attune the mind to the instinctive wisdom of the body. This tuning in to the universal wisdom of prana becomes a "tuning out" of all unhealthy preconceived ideas, beliefs, and tech-

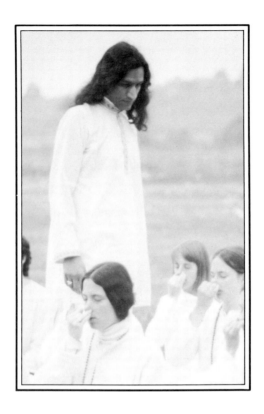

niques. Following the intuitive wisdom of the body gradually decreases body-mind conflict.

Clearly, the ability of mind to control prana is beneficial only if the mind's powers are used to support and then accelerate the impulse of this universal wisdom functioning through the body. Thus, we must make conscious choices that will allow us to live in harmony with our own body as well as with the body of the universe—Nature—which is our source of sustenance and survival. If, instead, we use our mind in conflict with the wisdom of the body, the free functioning of our evolutionary energy is inhibited.

Kripalu Yoga, by teaching how to attune the mind to the primal wisdom of the body, prana, assures the harmonious, cooperative functioning of mind and prana (or mind and body) that is essential both for survival and evolution. During actual practice this is specifically achieved by focussing the mind on the sensations and urges that are the expression of the wisdom of the body. I have explained this in more detail later in the book.

Fear: The Fuel of Ego-Mind

Ego-mind is our own individual creation. Thus when it is in conflict with the universal laws of prana, we automatically experience loneliness, separation, and fear.

When the ego-mind gives birth to fear,[1] the negative thoughts assume the form of emotions which are stronger than mere thought forms. When we practice body-mind harmony we tune into the universal wisdom of prana, which brings the opposite experience of fear—that of love, trust, and self-confidence.

But ego-mind has led us to identify so closely with every desire and pleasure, and every fear of pain or suffering, that we seek pleasures or guard against losses with the strong energy of our survival instinct,

---

[1] I am talking about the projected fears of the ego, not the natural physical instinctual fear which is a healthy self-preservation response of the body in the face of real danger. To be afraid in the path of a vicious wild animal is natural, whereas to walk the streets in fear of imaginary robbers is unnatural.

as if we were protecting our very lives. Thus our ego-mind easily dominates the superior wisdom of prana because fear is a more aggressive energy and prevents prana from functioning at the natural and the evolutionary levels. Survival level needs always take priority over evolutionary activity of prana, of necessity.

Fear created by the ego-mind through living against the natural survival instinct is even more aggressive and demanding than the survival instinct. As a result (in the unconscious person) fear automatically assumes priority over instinctive wisdom of the body. We have all seen or heard examples of this in people who would literally rather die than face something they are afraid of, such as someone who will commit suicide rather than face the pain of separation from a loved one. Thus fear can even suppress the will to live. This is certainly an extreme example, but we all experience milder versions of the same basic tendency in various forms throughout the day. So until we become conscious, we suffer from a hierarchy of urges: 1) strongest are the unnatural fears of the ego-mind; 2) next are the natural survival instincts; and finally 3) the evolutionary urge. So ego fears can dominate even the survival instincts, which in turn can dominate the evolutionary urge. Because we have lived unnaturally for so long, we are habituated to letting our ego's subtle fear needs take priority over our basic healthy survival needs.

Usually our energy remains clogged at the survival level, fulfilling the demands and protecting the fears of the ego. In order to experience the eventual awakening of prana, we must first free this prana so it can move up to its higher levels of expression. Because of this hierarchy of urges, we must first reduce the fearful thinking, feeling, acting, and living which stems from the ego-mind. Only then will we be able to tune in to the instinctual wisdom of prana in the body, and learn to again live naturally, which paves the way for responding to the evolutionary urge for realizing our higher potentials. This is the whole purpose of the mental disciplines of Kripalu Yoga.

Chapter Four:
The Practical Application of Prana Theory

Three Life Choices: Natural Unnatural, and Transcending Natural

Let us summarize how mankind has the ability to live at one of three levels of pranic activity: natural, unnatural, or transcendental. We are born with an animal body, a human mind, and a divine potential. Our human body is our natural self, our animal self. It functions directly in harmony with the natural laws, if it is not prevented from doing so.

Animals spontaneously live in harmony with the natural laws; their actions all come from instinct. So they have no choice but to live in harmony with the natural laws. All their activities (eating, sleeping, mating, etc.) are an instinctive response to their pure, physical, biological needs.

We as human beings have more than the animal body—we have the evolutionary gift of mind, which provides us the facility to either choose to live naturally, or to go against nature. When we use our mind to live in tune with nature, I call it "prana-mind." When we go against what is natural and healthy (wrong eating, oversleeping, overexertion, overindulgence in sensual pleasures, etc.), those choices are made by ego-mind.

When you go against your body, you go against the entire flow of the universal energies.

Our body is a miniature physical universe. Our individual spirit represents the Spirit of God. Our mind provides us with the freedom of individual choice and presents us with two directions in which we can go: we can go against the body, which manifests the natural laws; or we can act in harmony with the natural laws of the body, which will in turn lead us towards realizing our divine potential.

As we have seen, what makes mankind potentially superior to other animals is our ability and freedom to make conscious choices. But we cannot afford to forget that with the freedom of choice comes the responsibility for the consequences of the choices we make. This is the law of karma: "as you sow, so shall you reap[1]". Thus, we can either choose to support and accelerate our evolution, or we can move backwards and become even less healthy than the animals. Their survival and sustenance is guarded by the natural instinctive level of manifestation of prana.

Living Naturally in Body-Mind Harmony

When we attune the same mind to the body's needs and choose to live in tune with the natural laws—for example, eating only when we are hungry,

---

[1] The law of karma applies only to human beings because of the freedom to make choices based on intent, beliefs, etc.. There is no karma for animals because they act only instinctively, through the universal wisdom of the body.

sleeping when we are sleepy, choosing food that is good for us—that is natural living at the survival level, like a healthy animal. Animals lead a healthy life (unless they are around humans), but they do it unconsciously. To lead such a natural life consciously is the first step in spiritual living.

So we can use the mind to act according to our inner body wisdom (prana), or we can choose to go against it. But unless we follow the wisdom of prana, we will never be completely fulfilled, for deep within us we yearn to realize our potential to be one with our own divine source—God. If we fail to nurture our inner source, we are denying this innate evolutionary urge, and we experience separation from our inner source. This separation strengthens our ego and we experience fear and loneliness. On the other hand, when we act and live in accordance with the universal wisdom of prana, we experience inner peace, fulfillment, and contentment.

This is the whole inner meaning of the familiar prayer "Thy will be done, not mine, O Lord." It means simply that we live not according to our separate ego-mind but in harmony with (or "surrendered" to) the divine will as manifest through the natural laws, which are there for our sustenance and protection. This creates the basis for responding to and fulfilling our evolutionary urge. When body and mind are in conflict, it leads to unnatural living. To move towards the harmonious working of body and mind is to return to natural living. To transcend the limitations of body *and* mind is supranatural living.

In human beings, then, prana manifests in its

highest expression as mind and consciousness, and as a result we hold within us the potential to realize our inborn divinity. But before we can reach to the higher transcendental levels, we must first learn to live naturally again by using our choices more consciously. The whole purpose of the first stages of Kripalu Yoga is to teach how to reattune ourselves to the natural instinctive wisdom of the body. This returning to our natural instincts is the first step toward transcending them and achieving the supranatural states.

Our body is the foundation of life. Body can be mind's best friend because the body is closest to nature and hence more in tune than mind with the natural laws of health and harmony. Our mind is an extension of the body; it is the function of the brain, which is nurtured by the body. Mind is an evolutionary gift given to man as a tool to rise above nature. It has the potential to connect us to the most invisible essence of life, to realize the bliss of our inborn spirit.

Kripalu Yoga teaches how to reconnect with and respond to the natural urges and feelings in the body and thereby promote the harmonious and cooperative working of body and mind. By keeping our emphasis and attention on the feelings and instinctual urges, we become more and more attentive to the messages of the body. Kripalu Yoga also teaches us how to let the body guide our course of daily activities for sustenance, rest, sleep, and work, and how not to impose on the body cultural conditionings, habits, beliefs, and concepts.

Living Unnaturally in Body-Mind Conflict

If throughout the day prana is constantly directed to work according to priorities set by the ego-mind and is inhibited from providing for the body's needs—for example, if we don't rest, eliminate when we need to, or eat when hungry—it is unable to carry out internal healing and revitalization continuously, as it is supposed to do. As a result, prana can heal and rejuvenate only when the mind's control is relinquished during sleep, or in an emergency, for the survival of the body.

So if we constantly delay, resist, ignore, or only partially respond to prana's signals because of other priorities and habits, our store of energy is gradually depleted and our body suffers chronic stress, pain, and physical illnesses. This is what I call "body-mind conflict," the basic cause of unnecessary dissipation of the vital life energy of prana. This is what keeps us tied down to "survival-level" functioning and prevents our energy from rising to the evolutionary level.

The root cause of body-mind conflict is that ego tends to form habits of pleasurable and enjoyable experiences. These habits we store in our mind as pleasurable memories, and then our mind begins to crave more remembered pleasures and tries to repeat them more often. When we are totally blinded by the desire for pleasures, our mind automatically drives our body into unhealthy activities.

When such desires are in conflict with the body's needs and are repeated habitually, they create chronic stress patterns in the body. The body's toleration and resistance then begin to deteriorate, and we become more susceptible to pain and disease. This stress becomes localized into what I call "energy blocks" in the body, which continually sap our vital energy. The purpose of the earlier willful stages of Kripalu Yoga is to remove the physical blocks that continually drain the energy and prevent the free, healing flow of prana, and to establish a healthy lifestyle to root out the habitual causes of stress and disease.

In summary, we can choose to follow our inner body wisdom, the urges of prana, and live, think, feel, and act in tune with the universal laws of health, harmony, and evolution. Or we can choose to go against it, which separates us from our energy source and diminishes and inhibits the effective functioning of prana, the creative life force within us.

Living unnaturally in a state of body-mind conflict also affects us on the mental, emotional, and spiritual levels, as well as on the physical level. When we go against the natural laws of health, harmony and union, we develop a personality attitude that is separative, because it is in conflict with the natural laws. Nurturing this part of ourselves which separates us from the universal energies creates feelings of separation from other people, and thus of loneliness, insecurity, and emptiness.

To replace the inner union, harmony, and self-love that we lack, we look outside ourselves and seek approval, acceptance, and love from others. This automatically generates fear—the fear of not getting love; and this fear in its turn generates feelings of jealousy, competition, and comparison. Thus the separative vicious circle is completed: fear, insecurity, and inner conflict feed on themselves and continually increase.

This fear prevents us both from living a natural, healthy human life, and also from realizing our superhuman potential as divine beings.

So Kripalu Yoga teaches first how to return to the natural wisdom of the body, prana; and second, how to refine our physical and mental sensitivity so that we can attune to the subtler evolutionary messages of prana.

As we purify and refine our body, and are able to respond more consciously, we become more sensitive to the higher evolutionary urge of prana within us. We also begin to develop the higher, subtler levels of perception and comprehension of the intuitive and psychic faculties. Thus we can perceive the greater reality beyond the distorted and limited perceptions of the ego-mind.

For this reason, Kripalu Yoga Stages One and Two focus primarily on willful postures and pranayama to release the deep-set physical, mental, and emotional blocks. These blocks reduce sensitivity and prevent the healing energy of prana from flowing freely, and also sap our vitality and energy because they need prana for their existence.

Transcending "Natural" By Making Conscious Choices

We are born with mind and higher consciousness as well as with involuntary and instinctive functions.

In the hierarchy of natural evolution, human mind and consciousness is the highest evolutionary expression of prana that provides us with the means to go beyond nature. Mind and consciousness are like a sixth evolutionary sense through which we explore new dimensions of life: they allow us to understand and control the forces of nature and use them to our advantage, which is the subject of the physical sciences.

This higher consciousness also allows us the facility to go beyond the natural laws working within our body at a uniform rate. We can consciously accelerate our evolution through such techniques as concentration, meditation, affirmation, and visualization, which are the components of raja yoga. We thus have the potential of higher consciousness with which to transcend nature and thereby enter into totally new dimensions that lie beyond the powers of mind.

The beginning stages of Kripalu Yoga consist of willful yoga postures, pranayama, and other disciplines. By practicing consistently and with awareness, we become more conscious of the deeper and subtler messages of prana. This eventually brings about prana awakening, which accelerates the activity of prana from the survival level to the evolutionary level. It also results in the spontaneous, effortless "posture flow" and deep states of meditation.

Thus the benefits of Kripalu Yoga go far beyond the usual yoga benefits of physical health, to total body-mind-spirit harmony, which is the ultimate experience of the final spontaneous stage of Kripalu

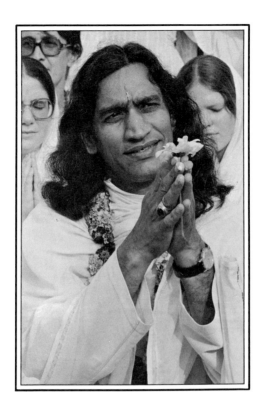

Yoga. This is the result of appropriate practice of the preparatory willful stages. Through this harmony of mind with the internal activities of prana we experience fulfillment of life. This is the true mastery of the art of living.

Thus, in addition to the physical practice, Kripalu Yoga emphasizes purifying the ego-mind so that it can more readily respond to the instinctual wisdom of the body and the intuitive higher states of consciousness. This establishes body-mind harmony so that mind works in harmony with the higher intelligence of prana.

Our body is rooted in our being. Our mind is not. We can survive without a mind, but we cannot survive without a body. And yet, ordinarily the body has no freedom to act independently of the mind except to carry out involuntary life functions, for which it depends entirely on the cooperation of the mind.

How to Recreate Body-Mind Harmony by "Purifying" the Mind

Our body is called the "Temple of God" because it is the foundation for the evolutionary expression of Prana, the Spirit. Our ego-mind, on the other hand, creates illusory limitations in our life that confine the expression of our spirit. This is precisely why ego-mind must be transcended in order for us to experience the divine dimension that exists beyond the mind. So in order for reality to reveal itself, the mind must be purified. But what does this phrase "purifying the mind" really mean?

What creates these impurities in the mind is all the accumulated habits, beliefs, social and cultural conditionings, fear, attachments, past impressions, future fantasies, desires, and dreams. These filter all our perceptions, interpretations, and interactions.

As a result, all responses to life that have been filtered through the ego-mind are not pure interactions but conditioned reactions. No matter how much we develop the skills of the mind, we still remain confined and bound by its limitations as long as it is distorted by ego. The mind is essential to our day-to-day living and is not to be ignored. But in order to actualize our superhuman (divine) potential, this mind has to be purified so it becomes transparent; its conditioned limitations and filters must be dissolved. So the true meaning of "purifying" the mind is to remove all conditioning which acts as a distorting filter of the mind. Thus we make the mind transparent so the light of the soul, of pure, objective reality, may shine through. Such an unconditioned mind is what yogis call "pure mind." It works in harmony with the Spirit—Prana.

In Kripalu Yoga this purification of the mind is carried out on three levels simultaneously, first by working directly with the mind itself through the techniques of concentration and meditation (usually only performed as part of raja yoga), and second by purifying the body through correct diet and the will-ful postures of hatha yoga. Our mental functioning is profoundly influenced by the physical chemistry and condition of the body because the mind is a function of the brain, which is an organ of the body. Third, the common foundation for these two disciplines of hatha and raja yoga is the practice of the *yamas* and *niyamas*[1], the ethical guidelines of yoga, for daily life, which help create both physical purity and mental peace.

A Summary of Prana's Role in Kripalu Yoga

To summarize: all that exists, whether animate

---

[1] These abstentions *(yamas)* and observances *(niyamas)* are nonviolence, truthfulness, non-stealing, non-possession, continence, purification, contentment, self-study, surrender, and transformation. See Patanjali (Taimini's commentary, pp. 220-252).

or inanimate, exists under the uniform evolutionary law of prana. In all living beings except man, prana functions only at the survival level and at a natural, unchanging evolutionary rhythm. Only mankind, with our unique gifts of mind and consciousness, is an exception to this law and can alter this evolutionary rhythm and accelerate it to attain the state of ultimate freedom.

The wisdom of the human body is the wisdom of universal Prana. Even so, we have the power to over-ride this pranic wisdom because our body is under the control of the mind. Even though this wisdom of prana working in the body is the wisdom of universal Prana, only with the help of the mind and consciousness can we actually awaken prana to its evolutionary level. Thus, mind gives us three choices: to accelerate our personal growth to a higher evolutionary level; to exist at the natural "survival" level which is common to the rest of creation; or to slide down to an even lower unhealthy, unnatural level of existence. For evolutionary growth, the power of the mind over prana has to be used appropriately, by teaching the mind to follow the infinite wisdom of prana working through our body.

Only when we allow the universal intelligence of prana to work fully within our body unimpeded by ego-mind, can it move beyond its involuntary and instinctual level. Then its natural wisdom begins to spontaneously accelerate the purifying cathartic processes which speed up our evolution.

Such an evolutionary awakening of prana is what

happened to me in the experience I described in Chapter One, when, without my conscious preparation or expectation, this energy started working involuntarily within my body. When my body moved independently of my conscious intervention, it was the working of prana awakened to an evolutionary level.

Higher evolution can be activated and continued not only through the medium of awakened spontaneous prana, but also through willful practices, both of which are part of Kripalu Yoga. It is important to understand the workings of prana, because although prana is always actively working within our body, this activity can be heightened when we follow willful practices. The deeper understanding of how prana works enables us to consciously support and even accelerate the purification and transformation brought about by the intelligent working of prana in our body. This energy awakens our consciousness to higher and higher levels.

So far I have only given you the philosophical principles behind Kripalu Yoga. For you to actually experience its transforming power, I will have to give you an understanding of how to apply these principles to your yoga practice and daily life on a regular basis. This I will do in detail in Volume II of this series.

The description of the Five Stages of Kripalu Yoga which follows is designed to first give you a thorough understanding of how these principles of prana's intelligence are incorporated into traditional hatha yoga in a slow and steady fashion. This gradually leads the practitioner to the final experience of

Meditation-in-Motion in which prana is allowed to function completely freely without intervention from the conditionings of mind.

Chapter Five:
The Five Stage Method of Kripalu Yoga

Kripalu Yoga is both very old, and very new. It is very old because it restores yoga to its original depth of unity, uniting raja yoga principles into hatha yoga practice. It is new because of the conscious use of prana in the practice of yoga (prana-vidya). From the very beginning the activity of prana in the body is the focus of awareness, and this provides a whole new dimension of awakening and heightening the evolutionary activity of prana in a gradual and balanced manner, in which the mind is not in strict control of the body as in willful practices, nor is the mind completely surrendered to prana as in Kundalini yoga. Kripalu Yoga is a newly developed approach in-between the willful practice of Ashtang yoga and Kundalini yoga; it is an approach wherein mind and prana work together in balanced harmony. In a spirit of mutual cooperation, mind and prana each contribute qualities to each other and thereby enhance and empower each other.

The Five Stages of Kripalu Yoga

Kripalu Yoga consists of five stages. Each stage roughly corresponds to a step of the classical Ashtang

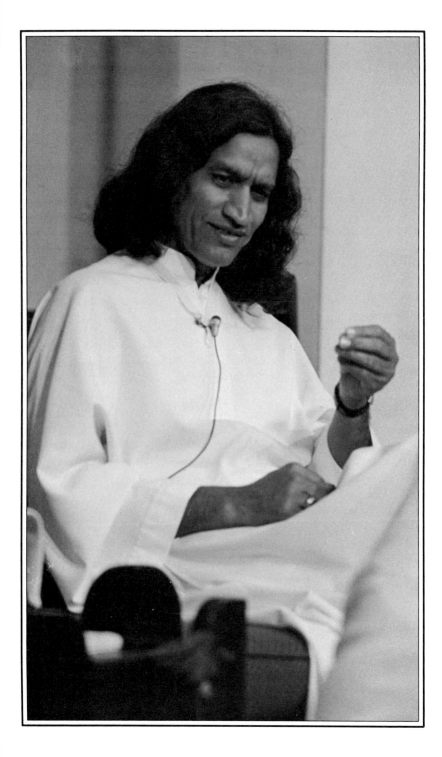

yoga of Yogi Patanjali. I have combined both hatha and raja yoga practices in the first four preparatory stages of Kripalu Yoga that lead into the final experience of Kripalu Yoga that is called "Meditation-in-Motion."

Ordinarily, stillness of the body is considered essential for successful meditation. But in the practice of Kripalu Yoga one experiences the paradox of motion (hatha yoga postures) and meditation (raja yoga) happening simultaneously. The meditative state during the posture flow is induced and maintained by:

1) deep relaxation before and during the practice of postures (asana).

2) rhythmic, continuous deep breathing which keeps the mind from restless wandering (pranayama).

3) extremely slow, meditative movements, which further slow down the mind and induce the drawing inward of the outgoing attention (pratyahara).

4) focusing the attention on the internal experience, and enhancing and deepening it through affirmation and visualization. This produces deep concentration (dharana).

5) remaining an uninvolved witness to all internal experiences and bodily movements prompted by the awakened intelligence of prana. This produces the paradoxical experience of spontaneous Meditation-in-Motion, where the ego-mind observes rather than directs the postures, along with a sense of effortless effort and choiceless awareness (dhyana).

When the body is profoundly relaxed, the breath is deep, slow and harmonious, and the movements of the body are very slow, the postures become effortless and spontaneous. In this state, the innate intelligence of prana, the wisdom of the body, takes over and the mind becomes merely a choiceless witness. The body is then able to respond to its own needs and chooses with extraordinary intelligence whatever sequences of postures, pranayama, kriyas, mudras, meditations, resting periods may be necessary to remove the energy blocks and tensions which create weakness and disease in the body-mind.

Stage One and Stage Two are predominately hatha yoga, corresponding to the traditional yoga steps of asana and pranayama. A major difference from present-day willful practices of hatha yoga is that from the very beginning the mind is trained to focus attention on the subtle sensations and urges that arise in the body during the practice of postures and pranayama, to develop a sensitivity to prana. This tuning into the body is tuning into prana, which establishes a body-mind harmony that is basic to freeing prana, because body-mind conflict creates tensions and blocks which restrict the free workings of prana. This lays the groundwork for later stages by incorporating the concentration skills necessary for raja yoga into the practice of hatha yoga. Thus the body is used as a tool for mastering the mind: hatha yoga is used as preparation for raja yoga. This has two advantages. First, the energy of prana will naturally go wherever the attention is focused, and this intensifies the physical benefits of hatha yoga. Second, focusing of attention curbs the wandering mind and conserves energy that would usually be dissipated by the restless mind. Thus raja yoga emerges quite naturally out of hatha yoga practice, instead of having to be learned and practiced sequentially, as is usually the case.

In the beginning stages of Kripalu Yoga when the mind is not yet completely purified of its conditionings and belief systems, and the body is full of blocks, willful formal practices as presented in Kripalu Yoga are most essential, and without them it is difficult to enter into higher stages of Kripalu Yoga. Kripalu Yoga Stage One and Stage Two focus primarily on willful postures and pranayama to release the deepset physical, mental, and emotional blocks that prevent the healing energy of prana from flowing freely. These blocks sap our vitality because they draw upon prana to sustain themselves. Some pranayama release old energy blocks, some are used to relax the body and calm the mind, and other pranayama balance and channel the released prana and help restore bodymind harmony. In general pranayama help control the body, prana, and mind.

Stage Three and Stage Four of Kripalu Yoga focus predominately on developing the traditional raja yoga disciplines of pratyahara and dharana, while at the same time deepening the practice of hatha yoga. These steps are practiced to develop control of the mind over prana. Thus hatha and raja yoga principles are interwoven throughout all four preparatory stages of Kripalu Yoga.

Stage Five of Kripalu Yoga is Meditation-in-Motion, in which prana is allowed to guide the body in an integrated holistic experience of asana, pranayama, dharana, and dhyana, all happening simultaneously. The fifth stage is the real experience of holistic yoga wherein the practice of hatha yoga is not separated from raja yoga. In the fifth stage, prana is awakened to an evolutionary level of functioning. The mind by this time is trained to attend to prana with such focused attention and loving cooperation that there emerges a unique partnership of body, mind, and prana working harmoniously together. This allows the movements of the body to be guided by prana, with mind taking a back seat and remaining a witness to the movements, though it can return to guide the experience at any moment if it so chooses.

Beginning the Practice of Kripalu Yoga

The intention of Kripalu Yoga practice is to experientially realize our direct connection with the divine universal evolutionary energy of Prana during our Meditation-in-Motion. In Kripalu Yoga I have adopted hatha yoga postures and pranayama as the medium for entering into Meditation-in-Motion. The earlier stages of Kripalu Yoga are to be practiced to achieve perfection of the medium, which here we have chosen to be hatha yoga. Just as Zen archery, aikido, karate, swordsmanship, other martial arts, painting, the Japanese tea ceremony, and so forth, are used as a medium for developing higher spiritual faculties, so too Kripalu Yoga uses hatha yoga postures and pranayama as a medium for spiritual growth.

The earlier stages are to be used to develop flexibility, sensitivity, and awareness of the body and to purify and remove deep-set tensions and blocks in the body to facilitate the free flow of prana. The earlier stages are also to be used to increase the prana in the body, which leads to prana awakening; to develop the storehouse of prana, the hara; to purify the body and mind; to bring body-mind harmony; to tune the mind to the body and experience the workings of prana in the body; to experience the relationship of prana to the mind, as explained in the previous chapter; to free prana from tensions and conflicts within the body and mind and to awaken higher evolutionary workings of prana.

I have explained the value of drawing upon the wisdom of the body, prana. This is to be realized in practice by applying the attention to delicate urges and sensations that arise in the body, and by responding to them. Sensitivity to the urges of prana and appropriate satisfaction of its needs is to be practiced in daily life as well as during formal yoga practice.

Kripalu Yoga is to be practiced 1) in daily life using the yamas and niyamas along with a simple natural way of life, and 2) formally using asana, pranayama, pratyahara, dharana, and dhyana, which are to be done individually and willfully, in preparation for the final stage of Kripalu Yoga, as Meditation-in-Motion.

Stages One and Two: Asana and Pranayama

The purpose of Kripalu Yoga Stages One and

Two is to learn the correct technical performance of the postures, to learn to control the breath and coordinate the body movements with deep continuous ujjayi breathing, and to focus the attention of the mind upon the postures and the breath. This corresponds to the steps of asanas (postures) and pranayama (control of breath) in Ashtang yoga. These two stages of Kripalu Yoga are a foundation for the eventual experience of the spontaneous posture flow.

Even though at first these initial stages may appear similar to the usual practice of hatha yoga, the unique prana principle of Kripalu Yoga is interwoven as an additional dimension of these two stages. From the beginning stages of Kripalu Yoga you are integrating the raja yoga counterpart into hatha yoga through developing concentration of the mind upon the movements of the body and breath. The basic purpose of this practice of Kripalu Yoga is the inner integration and union of body, mind, and spirit.

Attention is the key to the effective practice of the first two stages of Kripalu Yoga. The practice of Kripalu Yoga postures is unique in the way it brings together the usually scattered energies of body, mind, and heart into a harmonious unity. This is achieved by the technique of focusing the attention of the mind during the practice of postures. Focusing uses the principle of synergy.[1] Synergy occurs when physical, emotional, and mental energies are all focused together during the practice. Just as a laser beam is more

---

[1] Synergy: the action of two or more energies to achieve an effect that neither could do alone.

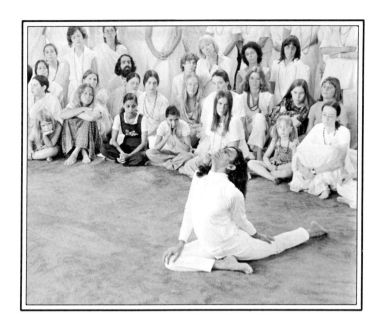

intense than an ordinary light that shines in all directions, so too such synergy brings about an ability to focus and control prana, which multiplies the effects of the postures manyfold. In this way, the prana is as totally focused as the mind is. This is an ancient secret of yoga not usually recognized or used. Mind tunes into the body through the medium of the sensations and feelings generated in the body during any specific movement. This develops a sensitivity to the body and to the universal wisdom of prana that works through it. This consciously and continuously anchors the mind into the body by attending to the inner experience through the outer form of bodily movements. This focusing technique increases body-mind harmony, reduces the restless wandering of the mind, and takes you inward into your own intimate absorbing experience. Since it is natural to achieve concentration through focusing, the practice is a more pleasurable experience. As a result, the usually wandering mind remains enchanted and focused naturally and effortlessly.

Various traditional pranayamas are also practiced to speed up the purifying of the body and develop control over prana and mind. Pranayama is used as a very powerful tool for awakening prana and storing prana. A volume later in this series will focus specifically on pranayama.

Stage Three: Pratyahara (Inward Withdrawal of Outgoing Attention)

The purpose of Stage Three of Kripalu Yoga is to learn pratyahara. Pratyahara is the withdrawal of the mind from input coming through the five senses. Pratyahara is developed in Stage Three by relaxing the body during the entire practice session and moving the body in an extremely slow, flowing manner. During postures, a passive mental attitude and deep relaxation of the body is cultivated, which, accompanied by extremely slow motion, automatically creates pratyahara. Usually energy is scattered and dissipated by the mind attending to the ever-changing stimuli of the senses. Thus pratyahara prepares for dharana (concentration) in Stage Four. The focused mind serves as a bridge between the internal world and the external world, between spirit and matter. Kripalu Yoga is the process of tuning the mind into the universal wisdom of the body, and when the mind is absorbed and the body is deeply relaxed you naturally enter into the witness consciousness, transcending the mind and going into the transcendental experience of Meditation-in-Motion.

Stage Three is pivotal in Kripalu Yoga. Through the practice of pratyahara, the senses begin to come under control, your powers of concentration improve, and the mind becomes sharp and focused. In addition, because the mind is focusing on pranic activity in the body, it develops a heightened sensitivity to prana, which prepares it for Stage Four. Pratyahara is the gateway to achieving mental control that will enable the mind to become quiet enough to observe and experience the flow of prana within the body, and sufficiently concentrated to direct the flow of prana in the body through the affirmations and visualizations of Stage Four.

Stage Four: Dharana (Concentration)

The purpose of Stage Four is to achieve concentration of mind. It corresponds to dharana in Ashtang yoga. The benefits are that the mind becomes concentrated and one-pointed through the process of visualization and affirmation. Visualizations and affirmations are given for each posture in a later chapter which is not included here. The technique of visualization and affirmation helps to accentuate the healing and purification processes integral to each posture.

Energy and attention are wedded; energy flows where the attention goes. Prana is naturally drawn to that part of the body affected by the posture, and focusing of attention there accentuates the process and increases the benefits of the posture manyfold. By directing prana to the specific part of the body affected by the posture, through visualizing and affirming, conscious control over prana is gained. As the mind becomes more and more concentrated it can be more easily brought into harmony with prana. When this occurs the mind will naturally become still. There will be an automatic expansion of consciousness and a profound sense of peace and tranquility.

In this stage willful mastery over prana is learned so that in the next stage prana can be allowed to move the body freely with its own intelligence. Prana cannot very well be allowed to move the body on its own unless the mind has first learned how to control prana. The conscious control of prana is a preparation for awakening prana to its own freer expression in the next stage.

Stage Five: Meditation-in-Motion

The purpose of Stage Five is to achieve a state of meditation through the medium of slow, graceful, spontaneous body movements that emerge from the body while the mind takes a back seat. The main focus of attention is attuning the mind to prana. This corresponds to the stage of dhyana (meditation) in Ashtang yoga.

After consistently practicing the first four stages of Kripalu Yoga, prana will naturally be freed and the practitioner will be able to enter into the fifth stage, in which postures are performed spontaneously and effortlessly as a Meditation-in-Motion. That yoga postures can occur spontaneously is an amazing concept for those who are only familiar with the traditional, willful approach to yoga postures. Nevertheless, if the earlier stages of Kripalu Yoga are properly practiced in conjunction with the proper diet, moderate lifestyle, yamas and niyamas (abstentions and observances), and right mental attitudes, this experience will arrive naturally.

The focus of attention at this stage is to allow the inner wisdom of prana to move the body—uninhibited, unobstructed, and unmanipulated in any way by the mind. At this stage, everything that has been learned from books, traditions, techniques, and authorities about formal yoga postures and breathing exercises has to be dropped. From this point on, one must learn to focus on only one authority: inner guidance. There is only one book you will read for the practice of yoga—the book of your body.

The preparatory stages of Kripalu Yoga remove energy blocks and tensions and deeply relax the body. This will progressively heighten sensitivity in response to prana's bodily urges. In order to be sensitive to prana, start with a few deep breaths and clear the mind of any need to achieve, force, prove, or compare yourself with others. Once you begin to move slowly into the Kripalu Yoga posture flow, keeping the body relaxed and the mind passive, tensions will progressively diminish. The tensions will slowly dissolve, and sensitivity to the body's own instinctive inner urges will become more and more pronounced. The flow of prana will become freer, and the body will begin to flow, move, turn, and twist, directed by its inner wisdom.

When the body first begins to move with inner guidance at the early stages of learning to practice the posture flow, the thought invariably arises, "Am I making this happen, or is it happening on its own?" If you continue practicing, eventually you will see more clearly the manner in which the body is moving. By and by, you will become convinced that the postures are flowing with great variety and in combinations that are unfamiliar, and that it is indeed your own inner intelligence that is behind the postures rather than your mind.

Any disturbance at the level of the mind will cause tensions in the body and inhibit the flow — disturbances such as indecision, conflict, need to prove one's self to others, need to seek acceptance or approval from others, fear, and restlessness. During the practice of the flow, one must remain established in primal awareness to respond to the urges of prana. This can be done only if one lets go of all preconceived ideas of yoga postures. Primal awareness is the state of choiceless awareness that responds to the inner wisdom of the body, prana.

Stage Five is the final and complete expression of Kripalu Yoga. During this stage, all rules and restrictions that have been willfully practiced in the first four stages are set aside. Instead, the postures are allowed to emerge spontaneously, guided by the wisdom of the body, prana. These may be traditional postures or even postures that you have never seen before in any yoga book. Do not suppress them if they occur, for prana is far wiser than any book and knows exactly what the body needs at that particular moment. Done in this way, yoga postures have a totally new dimension. They have become a form of Meditation-in-Motion, a prayer without words.

Kripalu Yoga posture flow is an effortless, harmonious, rhythmic and balanced flow of postures that produces inner stillness. The flow is guided from within in a meditative way that gives a timeless quality to the movement. As you smoothly flow from one posture to another, guided by your inner energy, you begin to experience a deep feeling of peace and stillness. In spite of the body's movements, the inner stillness grows progressively until you become completely absorbed in the inner music of movements created by the harmony of body, mind, and prana.

You find your own body making up new postures and new sequences to suit your own needs each day. The final stage is when you learn how to give completely free reign to the spontaneous inner urge. When the body orchestrates and choreographs its own movements, the movements are precisely and finely tuned to your inner needs. When the ego imposes its own movements or learned techniques, body-mind conflict is created that causes strain and stress on the body. When your attunement comes from being physically relaxed, remaining with an

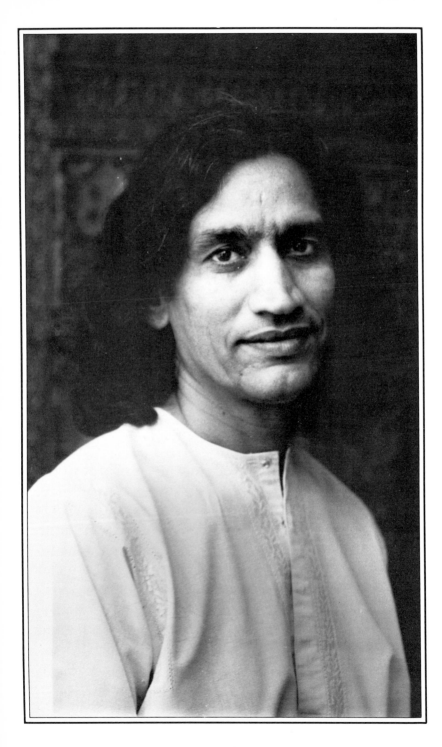

empty mind, ready to respond to the inner urges of the body, you are drawn into progressively deeper relaxation. Your attention is naturally drawn within, and the concentration and meditation simply emerge rather than being practiced.

Chapter Six:
Kripalu Yoga: A Rediscovery of Yoga's Ancient Origins

The Implications of Meditation-in-Motion for Personal Evolution

So, as we have seen, in the fifth and final stage of Kripalu Yoga, prana has been freed from its physiological and psychological blocks, and awakened to the "evolutionary" level where it functions at an accelerated rate of catharsis and purification. This occurs through spontaneous postures, mudras, and other *kriyas*[1], which happen without the mind having to know how to perform them, just as our normal involuntary physiological processes (such as digestion, elimination, respiration, and so forth) occur without our mind having to know how to carry them out. Both are accomplished by the same intelligence and with the same computer-like precision with which Prana controls the orbits of the stars and the galaxies, and the evolution of all of life on earth.

Not only that, these accelerated evolutionary

---

[1] Kriyas are involuntary cleansing, cathartic activities such as bellowing, postures, pranayama, dancing, chanting, laughing, crying, etc..

purification processes can happen to anyone who carries out intense physical and spiritual disciplines even without practicing yoga postures. This is how yoga was born, in fact, as a series of spontaneous movements directed purely by prana (later formalized into willful asanas), which occurred during the practice of deep meditation and other ascetic disciplines. This is why it is said in Kundalini yoga that once prana is fully awakened, no technical knowledge of yoga is necessary; everything that is needed emerges from within, carried out by prana's innate evolutionary intelligence.

At the usual level then, prana merely sustains life, whereas at the evolutionary level, awakened prana accelerates healing, rejuvenation, and purification of body, mind, and emotions. Not only that, it also awakens dormant "superhuman" powers, which are known in yoga as *siddhis* and occur along the way to the ultimate stage of *samadhi,* or union with the divine.

Awakened Prana: The Yogi's Secret of Power

From observing my guru as he reached to the highest stages of samadhi, I realized that when a yogi has succeeded in raising and stabilizing prana in the highest center of consciousness (in samadhi), he radiates his presence all around him in a steady stream of invisible, subtle energies that never fail to influence all those who come in contact with him. Such a yogi is connected to the unlimited universal source of Prana, and as a result his presence automatically nurtures all those who come in contact with him. He radiates contentment, tranquility, peace, and vitality, so that those who are in need and are ready can actually partake of prana and feel comforted, healed, revitalized, and transformed. They experience this energy of prana as soothing, healing, loving, caressing, and reassuring.

As far as I am aware, in Western culture there has been no structured approach or formal tradition like yoga that teaches how to awaken the wisdom of the body to a higher level of evolutionary activity. The techniques of awakening this wisdom of the body to an accelerated level has remained hidden as the wisdom of the ancient, mystical teachings of yoga. It has been developed empirically by the great masters of India over thousands of years and handed down to only those few, selected disciples who proved themselves capable of carrying on this most secret and sacred tradition. I was privileged to receive the secret teachings directly from a realized master, Swami Kripalvanandji.

Awakened Prana in Western Tradition

I want to point out here that this awakening of prana can be experienced by anyone from any cultural background, any spiritual or religious tradition, even without the practice of yoga, if they happen to create, consciously or unconsciously, the appropriate conditions for awakening of prana. I have read many stories of the lives of Christian saints and mystics in the West, in which they have had experiences of prana or Kundalini awakening without knowing it. One of the most easily recognizable clues is the reports of intense battles with increased sexual energy, which is an integral and natural part of Kundalini awakening. Unfortunately, because their spiritual tradition contained no understanding of prana and so no knowledge of how to prepare for and appropriately channel this energy when awakened, they reacted with fear and hatred of their bodies and what they saw as sinful sensuality, a "temptation of the Devil," and so on. Therefore, instead of helping this energy take its natural evolutionary course upward for further spiritual unfoldment, they chastised and punished their bodies with self-flagellation, hair-shirts, starvation diets and other penances to try to suppress these "evil" manifestations. So, sadly, the body was preached of as the "Temple of God," and treated as "Brother Ass".

So the power of this secret science of awakening prana lies not just in accessing it, but in also knowing how to raise it for the unfolding of the higher consciousness. As in the traditional spiritual paths, so also there are many modern cathartic therapies and growth techniques which use powerful methods that can awaken prana. Unfortunately, practitioners sometimes do not know either its true nature or evolutionary potential. Because they don't have this knowledge, often that energy is either suppressed, as the ascetic saints did, or wasted through familiar habitual channels which nurture the ego and the senses. Prana itself is neutral, but having more energy, awakening more prana, without discrimination, without knowing what are the intended higher evolutionary

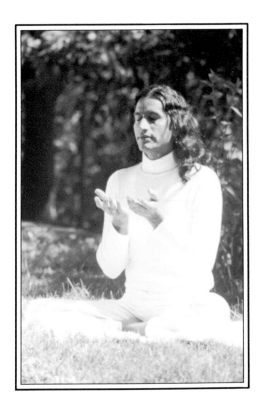

uses, can be very destructive. And here lies the importance of Kripalu Yoga: it provides a safe technique and clear conceptual and practical framework for understanding and channelling this powerful energy of awakened prana positively, that is, to the higher centers of consciousness, for spiritual unfoldment.

Kripalu Yoga Makes
Prana's Secrets Accessible

What is special about Kripalu Yoga is that I have adapted these ancient esoteric techniques of prana awakening and brought them into a form that is easily assimilated by Western seekers; and that I have tested it and taught it to thousands of students. Even in the early willful stages of Kripalu Yoga, people begin to experience quite dramatic energy changes. They report greater physical health and strength, more vigor and vitality, greater mental clarity and creativity, and feelings of love and compassion. It also opens to them a new dimension of intuitive perception that reveals the secret knowledge not visible through the five physical senses or conceivable through the reason or logic of conditioned mind.

This spontaneous wisdom of prana, which is the essence of yoga, has been overlooked in traditional willful hatha yoga, where only the external form of yoga, the willful postures, has remained. The benefits of prana are only received in Kundalini yoga, and since Kundalini yoga is so arduous, these benefits have only been available to a very few. If hatha yoga practices are done willfully and combined with techniques to free prana, they will eventually awaken prana. This is a basic principle of Kripalu Yoga, in which I have adapted these prana awakening techniques so that the many benefits of prana can be attained by anyone at even the early stages of willful practice.

So Kripalu Yoga is, in essence, returning to the ancient origins of yoga, which was born spontaneously from within. By practicing it, anyone can learn to again access this inner source of wisdom. So just as awakened prana was the source of the birth of yoga, yoga can become the source of prana awakening.

Without the full understanding of how prana functions at both the survival and evolutionary levels in body, mind, and emotions, the benefits of prana that can be obtained even through such graduated willful practices will not be fully attained. That understanding has been the whole purpose of this volume.

Internal Mastery of Prana is the Only True Mastery

The discoveries of the physical sciences that we discussed earlier represent mankind's triumphant quest for mastery over the manifestations of prana in the external world. Yoga, on the other hand, is a spiritual science which teaches us mastery over the manifestations of prana in the internal world of our body, mind, emotions, and spirit. Just as the understanding of the laws that govern the physical world gives us control over it, so also understanding the mysteries of these internal laws of prana gives us the true mastery of life. Through victory over the laws of the external environment, provided by the physical sciences, the most we can do is create a more comfortable life, a greater variety of pleasures, and more and faster facilities for enjoying these pleasures. No matter how much control we gain over the external environment, it will never fully satisfy us. Only internal self-mastery is truly fulfilling.

The five stages of Kripalu Yoga have been specifically designed to lead the practitioner towards that self-mastery in a slow and steady fashion through the mastery of prana, the life force.

Bibliography

Kripalu Publications

Desai, Yogi Amrit
    Kripalu Yoga: Meditation-in-Motion (1981).
    Happiness Is Now: Reflective Writings of Yogi Amrit Desai (1982).
    * **The Wisdom of the Body** (1984).
    * **Working Miracles of Love** (1985). *Collection of shorter works.*
    Love is an Awakening (1985).

Kripalu Retreat Staff
    Bapuji in America: Darshans at Kripalu Ashram (1979). *Out-of-print.*

Kripalvanandji, Yogacharya Swami
    Premyatra: A Pilgrimage of Love, Book I (1981).
    Premyatra: A Pilgrimage of Love, Book II (1982).
    Premyatra: A Pilgrimage of Love, Book III (1984).

Warren, Sukanya; Frances Mellen; and Peter Mellen
    * **Gurudev: The Life of Yogi Amrit Desai** (1982).

Books Distributed by Kripalu Center

Kripalvanandji, Yogacharya Swami
    * **Science of Meditation** (1977).

Muni, Rajarshi
> **Light from Guru to Disciple** (1974).
> **Yoga Experiences, Part I** (1977). *Kundalini yoga experiences; out-of-print.*

Books Available from Kripalu Center

Jnanadeva, Shri (Commentator); Pradhan, V. G. (Translator); Lambert, H. M. (Editor)
> **Jnaneshwari (Bhavarthadipika)**
> Vyasa, Shri Dvaipanya
> **Bhagavadgita** (London: George Allen Unwin, Ltd., 1967), Volumes I and II.

Patanjali
> **Yogadarshana (Yoga Sutras)**
> Taimini, I. K.
> **The Science of Yoga** (Commentary) (Wheaton, Illinois: Theosophical Publishing House, 1975).

Other Relevant Reading

Bernard, Theos
> **Hatha Yoga: The Report of a Personal Experience** (New York: Samuel Weiser, 1947). *Out-of-print.*
> **Hindu Philosophy** (Bombay, India: Jaico Publishing House, 125 Mahatma Gandhi Road, 1958, 1964), pp. 84-103. *Out-of-print.*

Besant, Annie
   Sanatana-Dharma: An Advanced Textbook of Hindu Religion and Ethics (Adyar, India: The Theosophical Publishing House, 1974).

Kripalvanandji, Yogacharya Swami
   Asana & Mudra (In Gujarati; 1967).
   The Sadhak's Companion (1977).

Singh, Pancham (Translator)
   Hatha Yoga Pradipika (New Delhi, India: Munishiram Manoharlal Publishers, 1980).

Tirtha, Swami Vishnu
   * **Devatma Shakti (Kundalini) Divine Power** (Rishikesh, India: Swami Shivom Tirth, 1974).

White, John (Editor)
   Kundalini, Evolution, and Enlightenment Butler, D. R., "Instant Cosmic Consciousness?" (New York: Anchor Press, 1979), pp. 184-188. *Out-of-print; included in* **Working Miracles of Love.**

* Recommended reading on prana and Kundalini yoga.

His Holiness Swami Shri Kripalvanandji

His Holiness Swami Shri Kripalvanandji (Bapuji) was one of the world's greatest masters of Kundalini yoga. For the last thirty years of his life, he devoted over 10 hours a day to the practice of Kundalini yoga meditation. As an example of his total dedication to this most arduous of spiritual practices, he missed only one day of meditation in this entire time—when he made his journey by airplane to the United States in 1977. For 22 of those years he practiced total silence, speaking only on rare public occasions.

Even though Bapuji was instrumental in establishing two major ashrams in India, his main focus was always his own personal sadhana (spiritual practices). Few truly great yogis have come to America; even fewer have chosen to come with such humility and self-effacement. After his arrival in 1977 Bapuji chose to live in seclusion at Kripalu Yoga Ashram in Sumneytown, Pennsylvania, founded and named in his honor by Yogi Amrit Desai. He returned to India in 1981, and entered Mahasamadhi (passed away) late that year.

A great poet, author, and classical musician, Bapuji spent most of his time when not in meditation in the activity of writing commentaries on the great

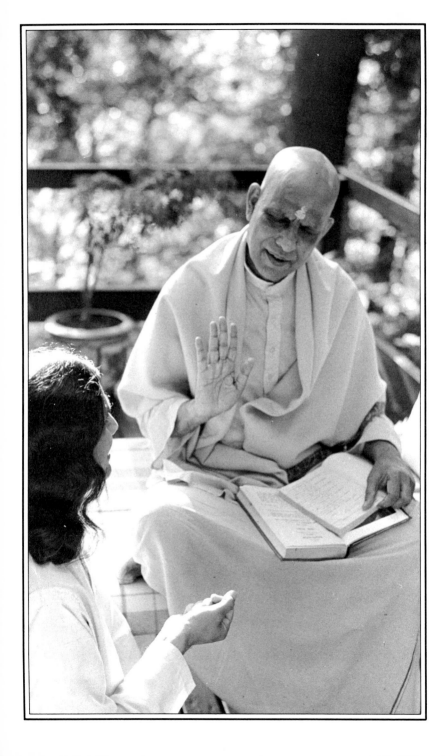

yogic scriptures based upon his own personal experience of the higher practices of yoga.

Major works by Swami Kripalvanandji that have been translated into English are listed in the Bibliography. Major works in Gujarati include **Gitanjali,** a poetic rendition of the *Bhagavad-Gita;* **Asana and Mudra; Hatha Yoga Pradipika;** and **Raga Jyoti,** a two volume work on classical Indian music. Books yet to be published are commentaries on Patanjali's *Yoga Sutras, Narad Bhakti Sutras,* and *Brahma Sutras,* all based upon his Kundalini yoga experiences.

Kripalu Center

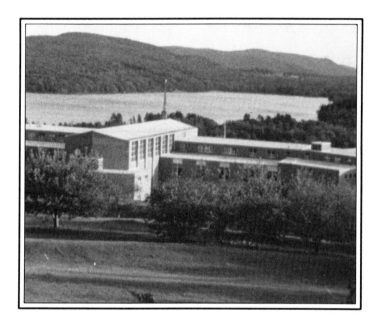

The fundamental approach of Kripalu Center is loving service to others. As Yogi Desai describes it:

> Our purpose is to help people, but it goes deeper than that. "Service to humanity" remains a barren, idealistic action if it does not also serve your inborn need to grow. If you establish the attitude that everything in the business of your daily life has the potential to teach you about life, then every experience whether pleasure or pain, success or failure, comes with a message that relates to your inner growth.

That orientation to spiritual growth has been the byword for Kripalu's growth. The present organization has evolved in its 20-year history into an independent non-profit federally tax-exempt corporation which is the parent of activities in Massachusetts, and also of a small, flourishing residential community in the original location in Sumneytown, Pennsylvania. The physical facilities of Kripalu Center are located on beautiful Lake Mahkeenac in the Berkshire mountains, in western Massachusetts. The main building, which has over four acres of floor space and 400 rooms, houses the resident staff of over 200, as well as program guests.

Activities at Kripalu Center

Yogi Desai teaches resident staff that true learning is experiential, and that we can only truly teach that which we live in everyday life. As a result, Kripalu provides both staff and guests a supportive environment which models the health and transformation principles it teaches. Guests may, if they choose, participate fully in the holistic lifestyle that has been developed over the years by the resident staff.

Group programs at Kripalu Center—weekend, week-long, or month-long—are educational and transformational in nature. These programs provide both experiential learning and practical methods for a way of life which integrates body, mind, and spirit into one harmonious whole. Guests, no matter what their background or work, can apply these powerful growth experiences to enrich their daily lives. According to their primary emphasis, our programs focus on:

Health and Fitness
Self-Discovery
Yoga
Spiritual Attunement
Bodywork Training
Month-Long Professional Training

Each program is open to people with all levels of experience, unless it is an advanced course in a series. As a guest, you may want to select a program that addresses a particular interest. Accordingly, we have grouped our programs into several categories depending upon their primary focus.

In programs with a focus on:	you experience how to:
Health and Fitness	promote your body's power to heal itself; move beyond unhealthy habits to a lifestyle which generates well-being.
Self-Discovery	observe and transform the patterns of thinking and feeling that condition your relationship to yourself and others.
Yoga	use the body as a vehicle to raise and center your energy; discard self-imposed limitations in body and mind and help others do the same.

Spiritual Attunement	invoke the wisdom that comes to you with inner stillness; draw upon this innate knowing for consistent inspiration.
Bodywork Training	activate your healing energy to enhance your own health, and help others as well, with a variety of hands-on techniques.

The daily schedule for guests includes three vegetarian meals, classes in yoga, relaxation, and Kripalu® DansKinetics, plus workshops tailored for the particular program. Private, double-occupancy, and dormitory accommodations are available; a program for children is open during the summer season. Guests and residents alike enjoy year-round sauna and whirlpool facilities, as well as hikes, swimming, or skiing on the spacious and beautiful 300+ acres surrounding the Center.

As a guest, your experience at Kripalu Center is a montage of discoveries: ideas and skills, facilities and events, feelings and friendships.

At Kripalu Center, guests experience what loving their whole self means. And that experience doesn't end when they leave. While they are here, they learn practical ways to keep that loving feeling going and growing, wherever they are. Freeing your self, freeing your love to grow: that's self-transformation. That's what the Kripalu experience is all about.

Yoga Teacher Training

This comprehensive training program offers detailed instruction in the theory, practice, application, and benefits of the Kripalu approach to the fundamental yoga postures (asanas) and breathing techniques (pranayama) that form the basis for living and teaching a yogic lifestyle.

Our training methods have evolved over years of experience and allow you to develop your own natural teaching style. Practice teaching, personal growth experiences, and guided self-reflection exercises are all included in your training to help increase your self-understanding and to enable you to communicate to those you teach with insight, confidence, and proficiency.

The month of training includes studies in the philosophy and psychology of yoga and in the teachings of Yogi Desai. Of special importance are the times spent in sessions with Yogi Desai when he is in residence.

You receive step-by-step lesson plans and learn how to tailor your yoga classes to special audiences and settings. When you leave, you will know who to contact and how to promote your services as a yoga teacher in your community.

To receive teaching certification, one year's practice of hatha yoga is required. Those not meeting this prerequisite may enroll for personal interest; their certification will be deferred until they complete one year's practice.

All Kripalu programs shift consciousness back to the body and highlight the need to balance energies and improve one's health as a prerequisite for achieving the peace and personal transformation or spiritual growth that is necessary for effective service to others. The Kripalu approach, truly holistic in nature, helps people tap their inner resources and lead fuller, happier lives. Living life as an art is the highest experience. As Yogi Desai puts it:

> When you consciously create your life, then you are an artist in the true sense of the word. Yes, I gave up my career as an artist, but only to practice the highest of arts: the art of living. To share this art with others is my greatest joy.

For more information on our calendar of programs, write or call:

Kripalu Center
P.O. Box 793
Lenox, MA 01240
(413) 637-3280